CYBERSURGERY

PROTOCOLS IN GENERAL SURGERY

SERIES EDITOR

Jonathan M. Sackier, M.D.
George Washington University
Department of Surgery
Washington, DC, USA

EDITORIAL ADVISORY BOARD

Alfred Cuschieri, M.D.
University of Dundee
Dundee, Scotland

Seymour Schwartz, M.D.
University of Rochester
Rochester, NY, USA

Kenneth A. Forde, M.D.
Columbia University
New York, NY, USA

Sir Robert Shields, M.D.
Royal Liverpool University Hospital
Merseyside, England

Lloyd M. Nyhus, M.D.
University of Illinois
Chicago, IL, USA

Robin Williamson, M.D.
Hammersmith Hospital
London, England

ONLINE EDITORIAL ADVISORY BOARD

Desmond H. Birkett, M.D.
Lahey Hitchcock Medical Center
Burlington, ME, USA

Carol Scott-Connor, M.D.
University of Iowa Hospital
Iowa City, IA, USA

David C. Brooks, M.D.
Harvard Medical School
Boston, MA, USA

William Stephen Eubanks, M.D.
Duke University
Durham, NC, USA

PROTOCOLS IN GENERAL SURGERY

SERIES EDITOR

JONATHAN M. SACKIER, M.D.

CYBERSURGERY

ADVANCED TECHNOLOGIES
FOR SURGICAL PRACTICE

VOLUME EDITOR

RICHARD M. SATAVA, M.D.

Yale University School of Medicine
Department of Surgery
New Haven, CT, USA
and
Defense Advanced Research Projects Agency (DARPA)
Advanced Biomedical Technologies
Arlington, VA, USA

WILEY-LISS

A JOHN WILEY & SONS, INC. PUBLICATION

NEW YORK • CHICHESTER • WEINHEIM • BRISBANE • SINGAPORE • TORONTO

Copyright © 1998 Wiley-Liss, Inc.

Published simultaneously in Canada.

Library of Congress Cataloging in Publication Data

Cybersurgery : advanced technologies for surgical practice / Richard
   M. Satava, general editor.
      p.   cm.—(Protocols in general surgery)
   Includes bibliographical references and index.
   ISBN 0-471-15874-7 (cloth : alk. paper)
     1. Surgery, Operative—Computer simulation. 2. Surgery,
Operative—Data processing.   3. Virtual reality in medicine.
4. Robotics in medicine.   I. Satava, Richard M., 1942–
II. Series.
   [DNLM: 1. Surgery, Operative—methods. 2. Computer Simulation.
3. Telemedicine.   WO 500 C994 1998]
   RD32.C93   1998
   617′.05—dc21
   DNLM/DLC
                                                97-17142

Printed in the United States of America

10 9 8 7 6 5 4 3 2 1

Contents

FOREWORD

This book is an eye opener. It is a clear and comprehensive account of the major technological advances which collectively will provide effective, high quality, cost-contained medical care that will undoubtedly become the norm in the near future. While the focus is on minimal access surgery, the impact of these technologies, *information, digital and display,* will be far reaching across all of the components of Health Care Systems. Indeed these new technologies will not only facilitate health care delivery, but also alter current medical practices by removing existing barriers between disciplines and by fostering the emergence of system-related multidisciplinary treatment groups in a low-cost ambulatory environment. Year by year, these hopes are closer to becoming reality. In producing CYBERSURGERY, Dr Satava has managed to recruit distinguished workers in the various fields who have produced, as expected, chapters of high quality on the component aspects, e.g., *human interface technology* which entails how we activate, interact, and control these complex systems; *advanced image display technology* which lies at the heart of all effective interventions and communications; *virtual reality,* the interactive pictorial representation of computer models or databases which will play a significant role in surgical simulation and in screening for diseases such as cancer and coronary artery disease (virtual endoscopy); *microelectromechanical systems* that form the 'smart' active components of endo-effectors, manipulators and remote sensing devices; *wireless remote relay systems* that enable Telepresence surgery, Telemedicine, Telementoring and Teleproctoring; *computer-aided surgery* to co-ordinate the output of various devices during complex interventions (systems software) systems that control master slave manipulators and systems for simulation in training; and *image-guided therapy* the percutaneous therapy with near real time tomographic guidance using helical CT-fluoroscopy, MRI, and electron beam tomography (EBT). The combination of real time tomography with surface viewing by mini-endoscopic systems will enable unparalleled precision in therapeutic efforts and scale down the size of instruments and smart endo-effectors to microscopic levels.

This book goes much beyond providing factual information and descriptive accounts of these sophisticated technologies which are essentially interdependent—it provides an awareness of the integrated whole; the various bits of the jigsaw puzzle have been fitted to provide an accurate broad picture of the shape of things to come. Undoubtedly there will be problems and issues that need to be addressed and overcome, not least amongst these are the ethical, legal, and moral issues which are described in a seminal and thought provoking chapter by Dr Kenneth Forde. It is often said that technology is neutral. While this is certainly so we must remember that its application never is, especially in relation to medical care.

I consider it a privilege to have written the Foreword to this book and have benefited and derived pleasure from reading the upcoming chapters. This book serves as a timely, unique, and important source of information which should interest all health care providers, purchasers, and planners alike in establishing the means for effective Health Care Delivery for the next millennium.

A. Cuschieri, M.D.
University of Dundee, June 1997

SERIES PREFACE

Surgeons are busy people, who are none the less driven to continually enhance their knowledge. It is that drive and the exciting developments in modern practice that have led to the birth of "Protocols in General Surgery."

There has been a dramatic paradigm shift in our profession; technologists have found surgeons and the two disciplines have thrived with the union. This shift in emphasis away from an art reliant upon simple tools, to a highly equipment–dependent discipline, demands a new means of communicating information to neophytes and diletantes both. That means is "Protocols in General Surgery," or "PIGS" as it is fondly known to those of us involved with the project—a catchy acronym which we hope will soon trip off the tongue of surgeons everywhere.

It is fitting that the first volume in this series should be directed to the very technology that was the genesis for this series, and inevitable that the editor for this tome should be Richard Satava. Simply put, no one person has done more to proslytize the new science—Cybersurgery—to his colleagues than Dr. Satava.

However, it is worth pointing out that the format for this first book is an aberration from the style of those which will follow, a fact made necessary by the nature of the content. We feel the reader should understand what we are trying to achieve with PIGS and throughout the series we will welcome your input.

The classic choices when putting together a surgical text are either the monograph—which suffers from being one person's view and from the workload and time demands that may well obsolesce it before it is ever published. Conversely, the edited multiauthor work tends to possess a widely diverse style, contingent upon the contributors. In designing PIGS we are attempting to have the best of both worlds. Each book will have a carefully selected editor who will glean opinions from "living references" and will then weave these into a sequential narrative, summarising where appropriate what is fact, what is opinion, what is fiction and what is an unanswered question. Selected readings will replace unwieldy bibliographies—we will trust our editors to sift through the corpus of published material and thereby avoid charging the reader for lists of papers that will never be utilised.

Recognising that surgeons today require Continuing Education Credits, we have arranged for CME to be granted for future volumes in conjunction with The George Washington University School of Medicine. As the science and art of Surgery is moving so rapidly, the series will also have an associated Home Page on the Internet, constructed in collaboration with an On-line Editorial Board. This is intended to be an opportunity for exchange of information, case presentations, research announcements and anything else that you, the reader, thinks appropriate.

At the risk of sounding like an Oscar recipient, there are a number of people who need to be thanked. First and foremost is Mr. Shawn Morton, Senior Medical Editor at John Wiley & Sons. He is the visionary who first saw this opportunity, honored me with the chance to work on the project and like an obstetrician, delivered the baby through a difficult labor. The Editorial Board has provided inspiration and guidance, in keeping with their senior positions in modern surgery, the On-line board has approached their challenge with gusto and invention. Of course, none of this would have been possible without them. They have all addressed the challenge of this new format with the thirst for excellence we have come to expect of people of this caliber. Finally I must thank my wife Shelley and daughter Chloe for their indulgence in allowing me the time to work on "Protocols."

We hope you enjoy this first volume and go on to read successive editions in the PIGS series, and also that you will let us know your thoughts—positive and negative—so that we can achieve our goal—to be the premier series of modern surgical texts.

Jonathan M. Sackier, M.D., F.R.C.S., F.A.C.S.
Washington DC, April 1997

Contributors

RICHARD M. SATAVA, M.D., F.A.C.S.
Yale University School of Medicine
New Haven, CT
and
Defense Advanced Research Projects Agency (DARPA)
Arlington, VA

JONATHAN M. SACKIER, M.D.
George Washington University Medical Center
Washington, DC

DESMOND H. BIRKETT, M.D., F.A.C.S.
Lahey Hitchcock Medical Center
Burlington, MA

BRUCE D. COLGAN, M.S.
Shadyside Hospital Center for Orthopedic Research
Pittsburgh, PA

ANTHONY M. DIGIOIA, M.D.
Shadyside Hospital Center for Orthopedic Research
Pittsburgh, PA

KENNETH A. FORDE, M.D.
College of Physicians & Surgeons of Columbia University
New York, NY

KAIGHAN J. GABRIEL, PH.D
Defense Advanced Research Projects Agency (DARPA)
Arlington, VA

FERENC A. JOLESZ, M.D.
Harvard Medical School
Brigham and Women's Hospital
Boston, MA

CDR. SHAUN JONES, M.D.
National Naval Medical Center
Bethesda, MD
and Defense Advanced Research Projects Agency (DARPA)
Arlington, VA

RON KINKINIS, M.D.
Harvard Medical School
Brigham and Women's Hospital
Boston, MA

NANCY KOERBEL
Shadyside Hospital Center for Orthopedic Research
Pittsburgh, PA

CYBERSURGERY

CYBERSURGERY

CYBERSURGERY: A NEW VISION FOR GENERAL SURGERY

RICHARD M. SATAVA, M.D., F.A.C.S.

Prelude: Star Wars! Cyberspace! To the public these words inspire visions of space ships, computer generated worlds and alien life forms, but to the scientific and medical communities these words epitomize the reality that extraordinary technologic success can be accomplished through selfless sacrifice and uncompromising scientific rigor applied to a bold and creative vision that dares to challenge the impossible. Efforts of this magnitude reshape the foundations of science and mandate a realignment of thought processes. When current vocabulary contains no words to adequately encompass these germinating ideas, it is necessary to resort to neologisms. Cybersurgery cannot be defined, rather it is a synthesis of this entire book, with the description of the individual technologies contributing to the meaning on a scientific, intuitive and emotional level. The reader must distill the essence of cybersurgery by imprinting their personal experience and interpretation upon these printed words.

Cybersurgery: Advanced Technologies for Surgical Practice,
Edited by Richard M. Satava, M.D.
ISBN 0-471-15874-7   Copyright © 1998 by Wiley-Liss, Inc.

I. CYBERSURGERY

The term *cybersurgery* is an attempt to embrace and describe a new conception for general surgery and a new set of terms by which surgeons can both comprehend and reimagine their craft in the Information Age. It encompasses both an emerging complementarity between clinicians and machines (particularly computers) and the integration of diverse digital technologies into the full spectrum of surgical care. On another level, cybersurgery symbolizes the recognition of a truly revolutionary era. Many authors have written about revolutionary times; however there are revolutions and then there are Revolutions. The first great Revolution in Surgery was in the late 1800's when the Giants in Medicine still strode the earth. Many names can be cited, however there were precious few visionaries who truly understood the magnitude of change and were able to give birth to the new discipline of Surgery. Among them were Bilroth, Lister, Virchow, and Moore. This disparate group never worked together, however it was the integration of their research and clinical skills which gave birth to the disciplines that made modern surgery possible. For it was the convergence of their visions and technologies that enabled Surgery, not a single event. Thus Bilroth brought the new skills and surgical instruments, Lister the asepsis, Virchow the pathology, and Moore the anesthesia. Without the synergy of all areas, modern surgery would never have happened. And in a relatively short period the foundations of surgery were laid for the next generation of pioneers to lead, the clinicians who exploited the technologies and advanced the art of surgery.

There have been numerous startling discoveries since these early beginnings, and many remarkable advances. These have been noteworthy in their own right, but none have changed the entire foundation of Surgery. The understanding of shock, cardio-pulmonary bypass and cardiac surgery, and transplantation have all had enormous impact upon the practice of surgery, but they have fostered the development of a new niche, splintering off a new specialty rather than change the very fabric of surgery.

II. THE INFORMATION PARADIGM

It is interesting yet obvious that the changes that led to the birth of surgery were contingent upon the discoveries that ushered in the Industrial Age. And just as the Industrial Age is waning, so too is the Golden Age of Surgery. The Industrial Age is being replaced by the Information Age, and conventional surgery is being replaced by a whole host of minimally invasive therapies and noninvasive procedures. Because we are currently in the middle of transition, it is unclear at this time how the shape of the next generation of surgery will appear, though the trend in the technologies are toward low power, miniaturized, low cost yet highly "intelligent" systems that will eventually transform surgery from minimally invasive into non-invasive procedures and whose development depends upon the emerging Information Age technologies which will be discussed in the chapters of this book. This is not to say that surgeons will no longer perform open or minimally invasive surgical procedures in the future, but rather that "conventional" surgery will recede to a niche, and non-invasive procedures will predominate. Laparoscopic (or minimal access) surgery is not an endpoint, but rather it is a transitional phase, between the radical approach of "open" surgery and the emerging forms of non-invasive procedures. But it was the advent of laparoscopic surgery that provided the "wake up call" to the Information Age, the realization that a revolution is occurring and that surgeons must extend their horizons to discover the direction of the future.

In order to have a revolution, all facets of the discipline must be impacted, rather than a single specialty. And a revolution must also reflect the same changes that are occurring in other scientific areas as well as society as a whole. It must be consistent with the global predictions that are proffered, such as The Third Wave of Alvin Toffler[1], MegaTrends of John Naisbitt[2], and most importantly Being Digital of Nicholas Negroponte[3]. While the former two authors gave us a peek into the power and magnitude of the revolution, it was Negroponte's concept of "bits instead of atoms" that brought the concept to fruition. He emphasized that what we do on a daily basis has, in previous times, required using actual physical objects (atoms); whereas the new technologies emphasize using information (bits) to accomplish the same task we had previously completed using the physical object. His classic example is that up to and including the Industrial Age, information in documents and letters were mailed physically from point to point (sending atoms across the country), whereas during the Information Age the same information is sent by fax (bits) at a much faster rate and lower cost. In translating this to the medical world, I will refer to "information equivalents", which are electronic or digital representations of real physical world objects or actions.

III. NEW DIMENSIONS IN VISUALIZATION

Surgical revolutions are, understandably, based upon changes in methods of visualizing the human body, its anatomical components, and the effects of disease processes. The first open surgical procedures, for example, required the creation of a new visual space for the "anatomo-clinical gaze," which now had to "map a volume" and "deal with the complexity of spatial data which for the first time [were] three-dimensional."[4] By contrast, laparoscopy limits vision and compresses three dimensions into two; while this "minimal invasion" of the abdominal cavity benefits the patient, who feels less pain and recovers more quickly, it presents a great challenge to the surgeon in terms of impaired depth perception and limited visualization.[5,6]

Advanced human interface technologies and display devices, combined with recent developments in 3-D visualization, however, will make it possible for radiologists and surgeons to create and utilize three-dimensional, "virtual," anatomic models generated from MRI or (helical) CT scans. (Segmented reconstructions of this sort are already being used to preoperatively plan for unusual or difficult conditions.)[7,8] In the operating room of the future, the cybersurgeon will integrate two-dimensional scan slices into three-dimensional images in real time and blend information from different imaging modalities to create unified video displays.[6] The surgeon will once again view complex body structures intuitively in three dimensions and "patient-friendly" surgery will become equally "surgeon-friendly."

IV. INTEGRATED TECHNOLOGIES

Transformations in surgical technology and technique have historically been the result of an accretion of effort and a convergence of discoveries from numerous disciplines, rather than sudden breakthroughs by solitary geniuses. The great revolution of surgery in the late nineteenth century noted above is an example of this phenomenon and it was awareness of the importance of the convergence of technologies that was the determining factor.

Similarly, the laparoscopic revolution resulted from the marriage of multiple existing technologies into a new art. For the first time, surgeons performed procedures without physically touching the organs they were removing or repairing. Minimal access surgery, the marriage of video endoscopy and laparoscopy, was embraced by younger, "Nintendo," surgeons whose innate haptic skills were potentiated by video games. The fundamental technologies underlying minimal access surgery, however, had been available for years: the fiberoptic light source was derived from the fiberoptic boroscope, an instrument used by every aviation mechanic in the 1950s to inspect the inside of jet engines; the charged coupling device (CCD) camera was first used in camcorders in the 1970s; and the laparoscopic instruments themselves can be found precisely diagrammed by Ambrose Pare[9] in 1523. The integration of these technologies was an issue of technology transfer in medicine: the result was minimal access surgery.

Cybersurgery is also emerging as the result of synergy and convergence as a range of new technologies combine to alter and transform the way surgical procedures are planned and executed, the architecture of the operating room, and the manner in which surgeons train and consult with each other.[10]

At the core of cybersurgery is the interaction of digital technologies to create an integrated man-machine environment. Eventually, the surgeon will stand at the center of a dense, highly interactive, information network. The components of this network will be synthesized into a system that is "natural" to the surgeon by means of human interface technologies and advanced display devices. Innovations in virtual reality technology will allow surgeons to actively manipulate and interact with complex, three-dimensional, computer-generated images[9] while sophisticated medical information is acquired, processed, and displayed by means of smart materials and devices, such as micrelectronic machine systems (MEMS).[10] Stereo imaging systems, computers, robotic manipulators, and microbots will combine to form a new framework for performing image-guided or computer-aided procedures.[11] Finally, the surgeon will escape the confines of geography to guide students or consult with colleagues via real-time, two-way audio-visual systems.[12]

Cybersurgery is the complete synthesis of these components, many of which are already in place, e.g., artificial intelligence, high-performance computing, and the Internet. As in earlier revolutions in surgical practice, the integrated whole is, and will continue to be, much greater than the sum of the parts.

SURGERY IN THE INFORMATION AGE

The cultural and technological forces that led to the birth of modern surgery were contingent upon discoveries that ushered in the Industrial Age. Most advanced technologies are now rooted in the

Information Age: products are etched in silicon and produced in the millions, rather than individually hand wired; goods are produced through "flexible manufacturing" and inventory management is "just in time"; virtual prototypes are designed and tested before any actual resources are committed; and, in surgery, a host of minimally invasive techniques have replaced the conventional surgical therapies developed during the Industrial Age.

The magnitude of the importance of the Information Age was revealed during a 1994 National Science Foundation workshop on Medical Applications of Virtual Reality, where the question was asked: "How much of what a physician does on a daily basis is really information management?" Using the most liberal interpretation, the answer is 80% to 90%. For example, during laparoscopic surgery, the surgeon looks not at the actual organs but at the video monitor (electronic image or "information equivalent" of the organs). When surgery is complete and the patient is visited in the recovery room, the surgeon glances at the physiologic monitor for blood pressure, pulse, and other vital signs (equivalent to the sense of touch). The visit is recorded on an electronic or computerized medical record (rather that writing on a piece of paper), filmless radiography, CT and MR scans, and other digital images have replaced films and microscopic slides, and surgical education is incorporating[10] computer-aided-instruction, multimedia, and even virtual reality for simulation and training.[11] Laboratory experiments in telesurgery have converted our hand motions into electronic signals, such that when the surgeon's hand moves, the electronic signal (information) is sent to the tip of the instrument, and the scalpel cuts—it's no longer blood and guts, it's bits and bytes. The importance is that in making this mental leap, in which the physician interacts with information as a substitute for physical objects, the capability exists to perform things not possible in the physical world. For example, by using Doppler ultrasound to display actual blood flows we can achieve the long dreamed of capability to "see into the body with X-ray vision." Exploiting the concept of "information equivalents" will challenge the reader to discover not only in this book but in daily practice, ways to extend both the capabilities of their surgical skills and the overall quality of surgical care.

The potential of this innovative approach to medicine can best be illustrated by the results of a "blue-sky" brainstorming session in late 1995 called "Doorway to the Future." This title of the sessions referred to how information equivalents tie together the fabric of medicine; it was inspired by many of the technologies discussed in this book, and aimed to integrate them into a meaningful system of complementary technologies. The following scenario was used to illustrate the future of surgery 10, 20, or perhaps 50 years from now.

A patient enters a physician's office, and passes through a doorway, the frame of which contains many scanning devices (like airports today), from CT to MRI to ultrasound to near infrared and others. These scanners not only acquire anatomic data but also physiologic and biochemical information (e.g., today's pulse oximeters). When the patient sits down next to the physician, a full 3-D holographic image of the patient appears suspended above the desktop, a visual integration of the information acquired just a minute before by the scanners. When the patient expresses the complaint of pain over the right flank, the physician can rotate the image, remove various layers, and query the representation of the patient's liver or kidney regarding the LDH, SGOT, alkaline phosphatase, serum creatinine, or other relevant information. This information and more is stored in each pixel of the patient's representative image (a "medical avatar") such that the image of each structure and organ (e.g., the liver) stacks up into a "deep pixel" containing all the relevant information about the structure. Each pixel contains anatomic data as well as biochemical, physiological, and historical information, all of which can be derived directly from the image and not have to be sought in volumes of written medical records or through a prolonged database search. Should a problem or disease be discovered, the image can immediately be used for patient education as the physician uses the avatar to explain what the problem might be.

Should a surgical problem be discovered, this same image can be used by the surgeon for preoperative planning or imported into a surgical simulator so that the surgeon can practice a variety of different approaches to the procedure before it is performed. At the time of the operation, the deep pixel image can be fused with a video image for use in intraoperative navigation or to enhance precision, as in stereotactic surgery. During postoperative visits, a follow-up scan can be compared to the preoperative scan by using image fusion and digital subtraction processing and the differences result in automatic outcome analysis. Since the medical avatar is an information equivalent, it can be made available and distributed (through telemedicine) over the Internet. Thus this single concept of replacing the written record (including X rays and other images) with the visual record of a medical avatar permits the entire spectrum of health care to be provided with unprecedented continuity.

Without doubt, not all of these technologies will be developed in precisely the manner indicated above, and many other technologies not mentioned will impact with even greater force than those currently envisioned. That, however, is not the point: The point is that we now have information tools that can fundamentally and totally revolutionize our approach to patient care; the tools that exist today are based on known and provable science. It is true that we must stringently and rigorously evaluate these technologies and concepts; yet we must not summarily discard them because of our Industrial Age preconceptions.

History is replete with examples of technologies that were available and ignored; it is imperative that we find those available today and use them, that we "think outside the box" and discover yet other exciting possibilities.

We must ensure that these discoveries improve physicians' abilities, rather than hobbling them with yet another technology

that will take a great amount of time and effort to master. The
devices and information systems of cybersurgery must be intuitive
and transparent to the extent that the computer or device "learns"
the surgeon, and not the surgeon learning the technology. Instruments should be an extension of natural actions rather than awkward and ill-conceived, like the current generation of laparoscopic
instruments. In the future instruments must be "smart," not dumb.
The coming generation of surgeons will be comfortable with Information Age technologies. To them, it is already natural to look at a
video image as a real object, or to use a joystick as a pair of scissors.
It is imperative that we play to these strengths, when appropriate,
and not discard an approach because it does not fit into the current
inventory of thought.

VI. THE AIM AND STRUCTURE OF THIS BOOK

This book is intended to provide a compact, but comprehensive, introduction to the technologies , techniques, possibilities, and limitations of cybersurgery.

Cybersurgery is divided into three sections:

Advanced Technologies. An introduction to the key technologies
and technological concepts underlying cybersurgery: human
interface technology, advanced display devices, and virtual reality.

Surgical Practice. An overview of how these technologies can be
configured to support image-guided and computer-aided procedures as well as telepresence surgery and telemedicine.

Ethical and Legal Considerations. An outline of the legal, social,
and behavioral factors that will affect, and to a certain extent,
limit the development of and application of new technologies
in surgical practice.

The purpose of this book is to provoke a sense of awe at the incredible opportunities that face us at this moment in history, a moment richer than any other in the past. Surgeons must use these advanced technologies described herein to extend their innate abilities beyond the fetters of the past. It is truly time to create the future.

We are leaving behind the Golden Age of Surgery, in which procedures were performed directly with the hands, and entering a new era when computers, micro-machines, remote manipulators, energy-directed therapies, human interface technologies, 3-D visualization, and virtual reality will converge to enhance both the manual and cognitive abilities of physicians through "information equivalents."

As we ride this wave of enthusiasm, however, it is essential not to forget our fundamental roots, our reason for entering the profession. Surgeons are first and foremost humanists, attending to both the physical and emotional care of the patient. We must remember that technology is neutral; it is neither good nor evil. It is up to the surgeon to provide the empathy and compassion that the technology lacks and, in so doing, to practice not only the Science but also the Art of Surgery.

REFERENCES

1. Toffler, Alvin—The Third Wave. New York: Morrow, 1980.
2. Naisbitt, J—MegaTrends. New York: Morrow, 1990.
3. Negroponte N: Being Digital. New York: Vintage Press, 1996.
4. Foucault M: The Birth of the Clinic: An Archaeology of Medical Perception. New York: *Vintage*, 1994:163.
5. Cuschieri A, Melzer A: The Impact of Technologies on Minimally Invasive Therapy. *Surg Endosc* (1997)11:91–92.
6. Seibel RMM: Image-guided minimally invasive therapy. *Surg Endosc* (1997)11:154–162.
7. Satava RM: Virtual endoscopy: Diagnosis using 3-D visualization and virtual representation. *Surg Endosc* (1996)10:173–174.

8. Rosen JM, Lasko-Harvill A, Satava RM: Virtual reality and surgery. In Taylor et al. (eds.), *Computer-Integrated Surgery: Technology and Clinical Applications.* Cambridge: MIT Press, 1996:231–243.

9. Paré, Ambrose: Apologie and Treatise of Ambrose Paré. Paris:1585, p151.

10. Satava RM: High-tech surgery: Speculations on future directions. In Sackier JM, Hunter JG (eds.), *Minimally-Invasive Surgery.* New York: McGraw-Hill, 1993:339–347.

11. New York: Churchill Livingstone, 1996:27–31.

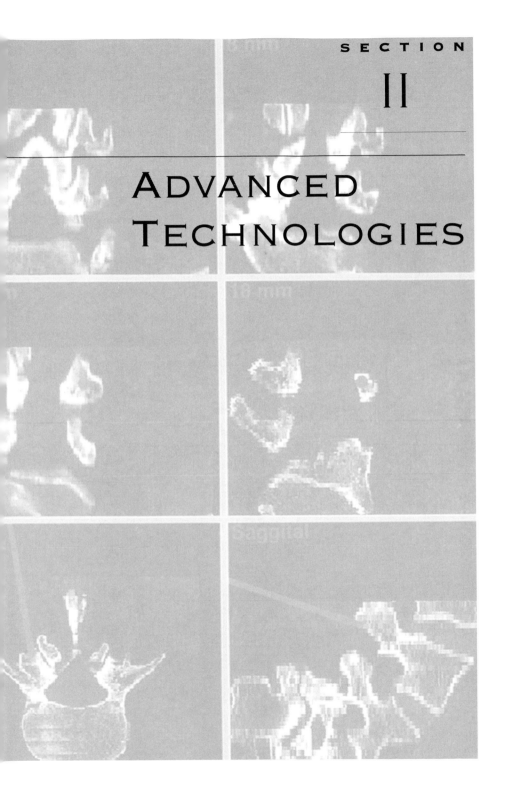

ADVANCED
TECHNOLOGIES

HUMAN INTERFACE TECHNOLOGY

RICHARD M. SATAVA, M.D., F.A.C.S. AND CDR. SHAUN B. JONES, M.D.

Human interface technology (HIT) has been discussed under many different names, such as man-machine interface, human-computer interaction, ergonomics, and so on, depending on what particular aspect is being emphasized. In essence HIT is trying to come to a natural and intuitive method of a person (an organic or biologic system) interacting with an electromechanical system (an inorganic- or physics-based system), whether that be a surgical instrument, an aircraft, or a computer. In designing such an interaction, there are two components of interaction, the input and the output. In addition there is the place where the interaction takes place, the environment. This can be a real or a virtual environment. For example, in a flight simulator the real part of the environment is the cockpit mockup, with all the switches, gauges, and displays, while the virtual environment is composed of the images of the terrain, airfield, or other aircraft through the cockpit "windows."

Cybersurgery: Advanced Technologies for Surgical Practice,
Edited by Richard M. Satava, M.D.
ISBN 0-471-15874-7   Copyright © 1998 by Wiley-Liss, Inc.

The input device is the device that brings the action or information into the environment (or objects in the environment which are acted upon); it is the efferent side of interaction. The output device returns information to the individual from the environment or object—the afferent side of interaction. Under many instances the input and output are part of the same device, such as in a surgical instrument where probing with a forceps into the tissue (environment) not only distorts the tissue (input) but also provides pressure back from the tissue to the hand (output). Under other circumstances, the devices are separate, such as in a computer (environment) where the input is the keyboard and the output is the video monitor and speakers.

The human is a complex integration of the motor and sensory systems that provide the input and output to/from the environment. As a generalization, the motor system provides input into the environment or instrument, while the sensory system receives the output. Anything that provides input is referred to as a *device,* while those objects or systems that provide output (to our sensory systems) are designated *displays.* Hence there are joystick and keyboard devices and visual, auditory, haptic, and other sensory displays. Not only must the input and output be designed to physically interact with the human, but the arrangement of multiple objects or information in the environment must be designed to provide natural and intuitive cognition and interaction of the entire environment. An example is the arrangement of the computer screen in the "desktop metaphor" first started with the Macintosh computers. Not only is the "point and click" of the mouse as intuitive as seeing and grabbing real objects on an actual desk, but the arrangement of the screen with familiar objects (icons) enhances the ability to use the computer.

While laparoscopic surgery has greatly profited the patient with decreased pain, less hospital stay, and quicker return to work, the interface has become an enormous problem for the surgeon. The surgeon has lost 3-D vision, dexterity, and the sense of touch.

The input devices (instruments) are awkward, counterintuitive and must move around a fulcrum instead of freely as in open surgery. The output received back from the surgical environment is nearly absent, with very little pressure felt back in the handle of the instruments. The video monitor provides a realistic representation of the interior of the patient, but it is a flat, 2-D surface that does not provide full perceptual cognition. Together these limitations degrade surgical performance when compared to open surgery. In addition the arrangement of the instruments relative to the monitor, patient and surgeon are awkward, the surgeon has lost the normal straight-line hand-eye axis from the object through the instrument and hand to the eye. Thus natural motions that were learned ever since playing with toys in a sandbox must be unlearned, and new counterintuitive actions must be practiced until proficient. Improvement in laparoscopic surgery can be made in all areas. The instruments must be designed to be less like standard surgical instruments and more like remote manipulators, which they actually have become once they are passed through the body wall and no longer directly visible. There needs to be sensory output back to the hand in order to feel the tissues as in open surgery. And the video monitor not only has to provide a 3-D image but should be located in such a manner so as to return the normal hand-eye axis.

One answer to the above problems generated by advent of laparoscopic surgery has been a number of "telepresence surgery" systems, such as those of Phil Green[1,2] and Ajit Shah of SRI international, Steve Charles of MicroDexterity Systems, Inc., Gehard Buess of Tubingen University and the Karlsruhe Forschungzentrum Institut, Russ Taylor of the Johns Hopkins University, Yulun Wang of Computer Motion,[3] and Ian Hunter[4] of the Massachusetts Institute of Technology. While each system has addressed the problems differently, they all are new and innovative methods of intuitively returning the "natural" relationship of the human with the real environment of surgery. All are mediated through a computer-enhanced interface comprised of input and output devices.

In the SRI,[1] Johns Hopkins, and Computer Motion's[3] systems, the surgeon sits at a surgeon's console that reproduces the normal hand-eye axis of open surgery. The image is projected in a manner that allows the surgeon to look downward (as if looking into the abdomen) and reach under the image to feel the instrument handles whose tips appear in the image display. Thus there is an illusion of operating upon an object directly in front of the surgeon using the "normal" hand-eye axis. In the MicroDexterity and MIT systems,[4] the emphasis is on enhancing the ability of human performance by receiving input from the surgical instrument handles and modifying them. By using a platform-mounted camera, moving organs (e.g., eye or heart) can be tracked so that they appear stationary on the video monitor; by scaling hand motions so that 1 cm equals 100 μ, precision positioning is obtained; and by using nonlinear filtering (between a frequency of 8 – 14 Hz), normal intention tremor is removed. The result is accurate positioning of 10-μ accuracy on the moving object, 20 times more accurate than the unaided surgeon is capable of doing. In the Karlsruhe system, the surgeon sits in a cockpitlike console, with the multiple video screens in front and the two surgical input handles suspended over the shoulders to precisely mimic the hand and arm motions. What is common to all is that the system has accommodated the surgeon, not the surgeon adapting to the system. (See Chapters 7 and 8 on telesurgery for full descriptions of the systems.)

There are a number of developing instruments that attempt to change the method of input to the real (operating field) or virtual (surgical simulator) environments. The previously mentioned telepresence surgery systems all have novel input devices (compared to typical computer interfaces). Some, such as the SRI system,[1] use the handles of conventional surgical instruments, while others such as the MicroDexterity system, are using modifications of highly specialized instruments, such as ophthalmologic instruments. The Karlsruhe system uses modified industrial robotic controls, and the MIT system[4] employs a highly accurate joystick device. The Johns Hopkins system is experimenting with a modification of the DataGlove concept by creating a DaumGlove, a glove device that accurately transmits hand motion to a three-fingered laparoscopic grasping instrument. All of these input devices can be used for operating on patients or for surgical simulators. In addition these devices have simple first-generation sensors that can convey back to the surgeon the sense of touch (see below on haptic displays).

One of the most important aspects of interacting with the real or synthetic world particularly in surgery is the visual display.[5] Ever since prehistory, humans have gone *to* their information sources, like the cave dwellers in France going to their paintings (information center) on the cave walls (Fig. 2.1). Likewise physicians daily repeat that same primitive behavior as they go to the computer monitors on their desktops to get information (Fig. 2.2). However, available today are lightweight head-mounted glasses (Fig. 2.3) that can provide the information at any place such as bedside, clinic, or operating room. An even more sophisticated development

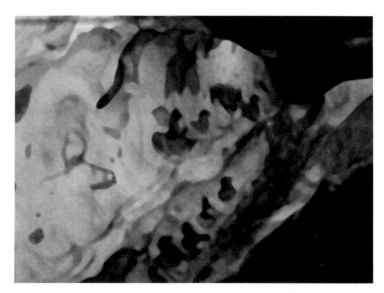

FIGURE 2.1. Wall paintings in caves in France.

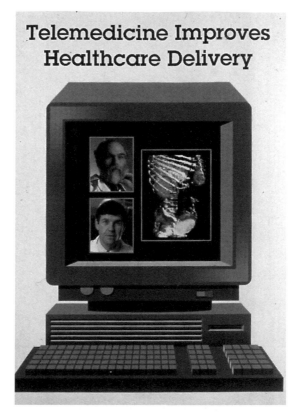

FIGURE 2.2. Typical computer monitor on desktop.

at the Human Interface Technology Laboratory (HIT Lab) of the University of Washington by Dr. Tom Furness is a Virtual Retinal Display[6] (Fig. 2.4). This is a tiny system with a diode laser that can clip on the frame of eyeglasses and paint the image directly upon the retina with ten times the clarity of conventional monitors. Or perhaps physicians will use a system similar to the CAVE of the University or Illinois (Fig. 2.5). Here Dr. Tom Difanti has created a 8-ft cubic room within which the three-dimensional images are projected; the physician would interact by walking between and around the images. Neurobiologists have been experimenting by representing the neurons of the brain and walking between them in

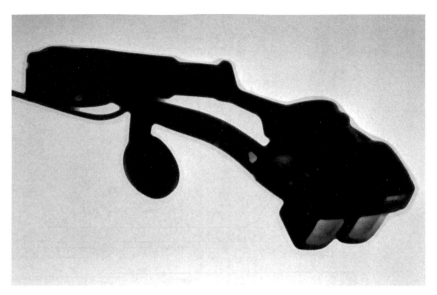

FIGURE 2.3. Lightweight portable head-mounted display (HMD) glasses (courtesy of Virtual I&O, Seattle).

the CAVE (Fig. 2.6); perhaps in the future we will take brain biopsies and walk between the cells to make the diagnosis of Parkinson's or Alzheimer's disease (Fig. 2.7). In studying anatomy, students could use the Virtual Workbench from the Fraunhofer Institut (Fig. 2.8) which portrays a 3-D image from the surface of a table top. In the not too distant future, many images will be displayed as a true 3-D suspended holographic image, as created by Dr. Jonathan Prince of Dimensional Media Associates[7] (Fig. 2.9). These images are actually suspended in free space such that a hand can pass directly through them, or if a haptic input device is used, the textures, surfaces and even pulsatile motions can be felt. Most of these technologies are in early versions or prototypes, and it is uncertain which will ultimately be used. However, the variety of visual displays ensures that entirely new methods of interacting with images can provide a richer opportunity to optimize information about patients and that their use will not be determined by the technology but by the creative applications these opportunities offer.

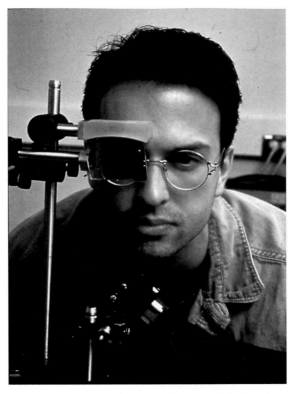

FIGURE 2.4. Virtual retinal display (VRD) in early benchtop prototype (courtesy Dr. Tom Furness, HIT Lab, Seattle).

The output from the environment back to other sensory displays is not as sophisticated or developed as the visual displays. Areas where advances have occurred are acoustic (sound) and haptic (touch and position). There are preliminary investigations in smell by Myron Kruger[8] but without any currently working prototypes, and there are no displays for taste.

The area of 3-D sound has been investigated by Scott Foster and Beth Wensel, with the baseline 3-D acoustic system called Convolvotron first developed under NASA sponsorship in the late 1980s. The primary strength of the system is to provide acoustic spatial localization. Because of binaural hearing, the human is capable of accurately localizing the position of the source of a sound in

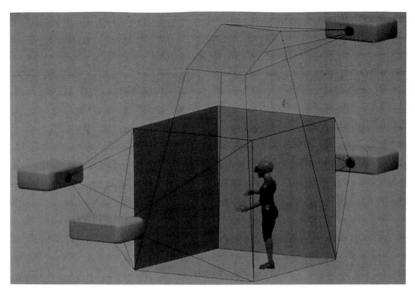

FIGURE 2.5. The CAVE environment, with illustration of person within the 8-ft cubic room and images projected (courtesy Dr. Tom Defanti, University of Illinois, Chicago).

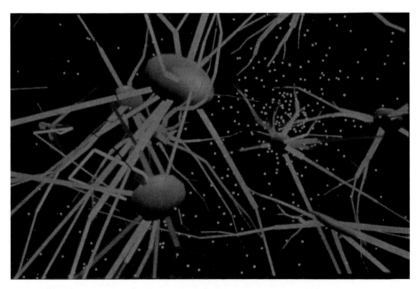

FIGURE 2.6. Graphic representations of brain cells the size of footballs and neurons for display in the CAVE (courtesy Dr. Tom Defanti, University of Illinois, Chicago).

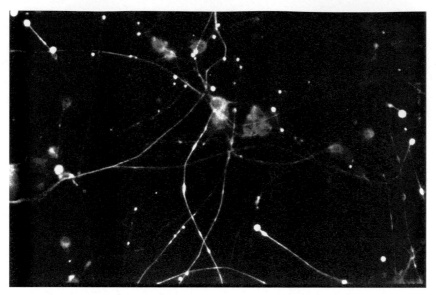

FIGURE 2.7. Histologic image of a brain biopsy (courtesy Dr. Brian Athey, University of Michigan, Ann Arbor).

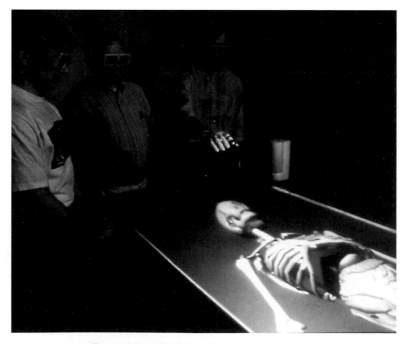

FIGURE 2.8. Responsive Workbench with a virtual cadaver (courtesy of Fraunhofer Institut, Stuttgart).

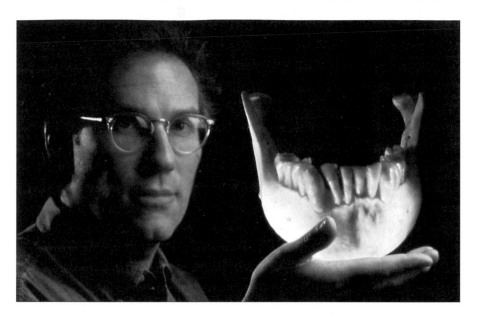

FIGURE 2.9. Suspended 3-D holographic image of a mandible (courtesy of Jonathan Prince, Dimensional Media Associates, New York).

the environment; however, the question is how will this capability be applicable for surgical practice—there are no proposed uses at this time. Presently Professor Dan Karron of New York University is investigating the use of sound to aid in accurate positioning of surgical instruments within the operating field. As an instrument comes closer to an intended structure or target, the intensity, frequency, pitch, and quality of sound can increase to give an added sensory cue that would assist in determining proximity to the object. In microsurgery where the forces of contact are at or below the threshold of human perception, the use of sound can be added to indicate the amount of force the surgeon is either applying or receiving. The substitution of one sensory modality (in this case, touch) with a different modality (sound) is referred to as *synesthesia*; it is a method of enhancing our skills and capabilities. As these new explorations in synesthesia develop, it will be up to the practicing clinical surgeon to help determine where these new capabilities can best be implemented.

The haptic input devices have had a decade or more of serious investigation,[9] and there are a few commercial products available, mainly in virtual environments for simulation. The sense of touch is an enormously complex system, and for practical purposes (as applied to surgical systems or simulators) it has two main components: the force component to feel the pressure back on the hand or fingers, and the tactile component to give the sense of texture and shape to the fingertips. (This description ignores the other components of proprioception, vibration, temperature, kinesthesia, etc.) While this is not an accurate scientific description, it provides a convenient oversimplified method of understanding the complexity of displaying what is generally referred to as touch. The Immersion Probe and the Phantom are two commercial devices, and Dr. Greg Burdea[10] has a very sophisticated glove-based device that can provide force reflection feedback for the sense of pressure back to the hand and fingers. These are purely mechanical devices, not too dissimilar in function from a joystick, that "pushes back" when either the remote manipulator touches a real object or the imaginary instrument in a simulation touches the surface of the imaginary tissue or organ. Thus, by the resistance the device provides, the surgeon "feels" the edges and consistency of the object. The systems can be adapted to use any number of different devices to be held, such as a thimble to feel the surfaces and edges or objects, or actual surgical instruments, probes, or needles (to practice a spinal tap, biopsy, or IV insertion) to perform specific procedures. In order to feel very subtle changes such as surface texture, the slipping and sliding of tissue between the fingers, and so on, the device must provide a display to the small surface of the fingertip pads. Numerous attempts are occurring at this time, from very small arrays of pins that poke a particular pattern on the fingertip, to balloon devices, to highly localized vibratory systems. While these are all interesting, there is none to date that comes close to reproducing the full dynamic range of our tactile sensation, let alone incorporation into a commercial product. It is important to note that all the telesurgery systems are employing some form of haptic display that is proprietary to a particular system.

While we have all the above-illustrated technological approaches for optimal interfaces, one of the key issue for the future of medicine will be how we represent the information about our patients by using the principles of human interface technology. While the litany of different visual displays provides ample opportunities, one promising concept is to represent the patient as a virtual 3-D holographic object. Recent advances in 3-D visualization and reconstruction from CT, MRI, and ultrasound images now have the ability to recreate a full volumetric representation of the patient—a medical avatar. (Avatar comes from medieval literature and modern video games. Ancient mythology referred to the representations such as lions, dragons, or handsome princes which wizards transformed into as avatars; in today's video games the avatar is the image that appears in the game as the stand-in representation of the person playing the game.) Not only can the avatar be anatomically correct, but if other data are added to the image from functional, physical characteristics, biochemical, or physiologic parameters, then the avatar will contain real data representing the current state of the patient. Since the image is comprised of millions of pixels (which are data points that describe the location and position of each organ or tissue), using sophisticated techniques of "data fusion," the other appropriate parameters can be added to each pixel. Thus, for example, the liver of the avatar would not only have information about its size, shape, color, and texture but also the elasticity and strength of the parenchyma (should it be "cut"), the Doppler flow rate of the portal vein, and the value of the SGOT, LDH, alkaline phosphatase, and other biochemical values. Conceptually we are stacking up in each pixel information about every organ and tissue in the body, creating "deep pixels" which provide the same information as the patient's medical chart would normally provide—in essence a visual database about the patient. And just as an infant or young child handles and touches objects in the world to learn about them, it would be possible to use a haptic input device to "touch" the avatar and receive all the information about the particular organ or tissue. This information would be not only a vertical record (i.e., all the information about the patient, including historical information, e.g., allergies and past surgery) but also a continuous horizontal record to ensure the full spectrum of medical care. The avatar could be used to show the patient precisely what is the problem or disease. It could be used to plan a specific operation or be imported into a surgical simulator to practice a number of different approaches to a surgical operation. During surgery, by using data fusion with the video or radiologic image of the patient, it could aid in surgical navigation. Following surgery, a repeat set of studies could be performed and compared to preoperative avatar, using data fusion and digital subtraction for accurate outcomes analysis. Hence this would provide continuity of the full spectrum of health care using a single image.

In Nicholas Negroponte's book "Being Digital"[11] there are repeated references to the potential directions that the human interface can go. The underlying principles continue to revolve around an interface, which is intuitive, unencumbering, transparent, intelligent, and anticipatory. Intuitive is used in the sense that during the interaction, it is obvious what must be done or meant (like the icon on a desk-top metaphor in which a file folder is where you file documents)—no instructions are required. Transparent means that the person is not thinking that they are giving a command to the computer (such as typing in instructions on a computer program), rather the action has the impression of doing a natural act of pointing at what is desired. There are no truly transparent interfaces today except voice recognition and command: When a person wants something, they just talk as if they were giving a request or command to another person. Unencumbering refers to how awkward and intrusive the device that is used for the interface is; HMDs are very uncomfortable and obstructive of vision, whereas the handles of a telesurgery system that are identical to surgical tools are not.

Intelligent describes the ability of the system to fully understand the intentions of the person, and automatically accommodates for any possible misunderstandings—there are computer programs that can tell the difference in the spoken word between to, too, and two, depending upon the context and grammar structure in which it is spoken. Anticipatory is being reflected in the new "agents" that are appearing on the browsers of the World Wide Web; the brower "watches" the different subjects you search when you surf the web, and the next time you are ready to search, the browser already has a list of all the information in the areas which you routinely search. More sophisticated versions now monitor many functions and collate the information; when a phone call arrives it determines who the caller is, checks the scheduler to see if the caller has an appointment, searches the letter file for recent correspondence, checks the financial database for any billing, and then presents all that information at the time the call is being transferred to the person. Negroponte uses the analogy of the ideal interface being a personal butler for everyone; it knows your past associations, habits, schedule, individual likes and dislikes and even your choice of food and provides whatever it is that you want (and probably need but forgot to ask for) in a timely fashion. We are not there yet, however the underlying points apply to all areas where humans interact in their environment. We must design our technologies in such a fashion that the interfaces are always smart, so that the device, computer or instrument learns us rather than we learning them. This will empower the individual to perform more efficiently and effectively, and in so doing, provide a much higher quality of health care.

REFERENCES

1. Green PS, Hill JH, and Satava RM. Telepresence: Dextrous procedures in a virtual operating field. (Abstr). *Surg Endosc* 57:192, 1991

2. Green PS, Hill JW, Jensen JF, and Shah A. Telepresence Surgery. *IEEE Engineering in Medicine in Biology* 14:324–29, 1995.

3. Wang Y. A Clinical Examination of Robotics in Surgery. *Jour of Med and Virtual Reality* accepted for publication.

4. Hunter IW, Doukoglou TD, Lafontaine SR, et al. A Teleoperated Microsurgical Robot and Associated Virtual Environment for Eye Surgery. *Presence* 4:265–80, 1993.

5. Cuschieri A. Visual Displays and Visual Perception in Minimal Access Surgery. *Seminars in Laparoscopic Surgery* 2:209–14, 1995.

6. Barfield W and Furness TA. Virtual Environments and Advanced Interface Design. New York, Oxford University Press (1995)

7. Chinnock C. Holographic 3-D Images float in free space. *Laser Focus World* June 1995 pp 22–24.

8. Kruger MW. Olfactory Stimuli in Virtual Reality Applications, pp 180–81. In Satava RM, Morgan K, et al *Interactive Technology and the New Medical Paradigm for Health Care.* IOS Press: Washington, 1995.

9. Salisbury JK, Brock D, Massie T, Swarup N, and Zilles C. Haptic rendering: Programming touch interaction with virtual objects *Proc of ACM 1995 Symposium on Interactive 3-D Graphics* Monterey CA, April 1995.

10. Burdea G and Coifett P. Touch and Force Feedback Chapter 3 pp, 81–116 in *Virtual Reality Technology,* New York: John Wiley & Sons, Inc. 1994.

11. Negroponte N. Being Digital. New York: Vintage Press, 1996.

ADVANCED DISPLAY DEVICES

DESMOND H. BIRKETT, M.D., F.A.C.S.

I. INTRODUCTION

From its inception by Georg Kelling in 1901, until recently, laparoscopy has been carried out by direct applying the eye to a rigid
laparoscope to view the inside of the abdominal cavity.[1] However,
as a result of advances in the technology of imaging, particularly
the introduction of small, lightweight video cameras with low-light
capabilities that can display a good quality image on a video monitor, the scope of laparoscopy for the general surgeon has been
opened up and resulted in the introduction of therapeutic laparoscopy. These changes arising from the new technology have distinct advantages over the older direct visual laparoscopy. They permit the surgeon to use both hands to perform a therapeutic
procedure rather than needing one hand to hold the laparoscope. It
also makes it easier to have one or more assistants rather than the
older method of an assistant looking through a side-arm eyepiece
from a beam splitter. More people in the operating room can see
the operation on the monitor and follow its performance by the

Cybersurgery: Advanced Technologies for Surgical Practice,
Edited by Richard M. Satava, M.D.
ISBN 0-471-15874-7   Copyright © 1998 by Wiley-Liss, Inc.

surgeon and assistant, and that allows the scrub nurse to be part of the operation and anticipate the instruments likely to be needed. It is certainly less tiring for the surgeon and assistant to view a monitor than directly looking through an instrument. However, there are limitations to this new method of visualization. It is an electronic reconstruction of the view at the end of the endoscope, with the colors adjusted by the observer to a level that he or she feels represents the situation within the abdomen. This image is then displayed on a video monitor with its inherent good, but not excellent, image reproduction. There are other problems with this technology, there is the compromise of peripheral vision which can be a severe limitation when the instruments are moved out of the field of view. Bearing in mind these limitations, the current two-dimensional charged coupled device (CCD) cameras, either the two- or three-chip cameras, have excellent resolution and low-light capacity making fine manipulative procedures easy to perform. Performance of these tasks will become easier with the much needed further improvement in imaging technology and the possible wider use of three-dimensional imaging.

The current display screens are anything but perfect, and they require significant improvement. The current cathode ray tube (CRT) screens are bulky and, because of their size, often have to be placed off to the side and not in front of the surgeon. This means that to view the image at the end of the instruments that are being manipulated, the surgeon is not looking in the line of his/her hands and may have to intermittently look around an assistant's head that gets in the way of the poorly placed monitor, or he/she may be distracted by what is going on around the monitor, interfering with his/her concentration. As a result of the poorly positioned monitor the observer's head may be turned to the side, resulting in discomfort and neck ache during a long procedure. The resolution on the current monitors, although good, may at times be less than totally acceptable.

II. VIDEO CAMERAS

The early video cameras, which were saticon tube cameras, were bulky, heavy, and cumbersome. Their light sensitivity was poor as was the resolution, which made their use suboptimal for laparoscopic procedures. The introduction of the CCD cameras was a major advance because these cameras were small, lightweight, and with good low-light sensitivity. It is these characteristics that have made their use possible in laparo-endoscopic procedures. This change resulted in the rapid growth of laparoscopy in the early 1990s. The initial CCD cameras were single chips with filters in front of the chip for the three primary colors. The technology has improved, resulting in the production of the current-day cameras with low-light sensitivity and excellent resolution. The color resolution has improved with the introduction of the three-chip cameras, with one chip for each primary color. The three-chip technology has improved both the definition and the color of the images, giving a clearer image with better resolution.

These single or three-chip CCD cameras come more commonly as separate units that can be attached to laparoscopes of varying sizes, from 2 to 10 mm in diameter with varying angulation of the distal end from 0 to 40 degrees. These detachable units have both advantages and disadvantages. The detachable nature of the camera increases the versatility of the system because of the number of instruments to which it can be attached; however, the connection means a glass-air-glass interface which reduces the light-carrying capacity of the system and the potential for water condensation on the glass surfaces causing interference with the image quality. These problems can be overcome with an integral unit in which the camera is fused onto the top of the laparoscope as one unit. These units are smaller and lighter in weight and have better light transmission, but with the majority of systems the laparoscope and camera must be changed, if an angled laparoscope is needed during a procedure, and the new camera readjusted. These systems are more expensive than the detachable combinations. There is a distinct advantage to only changing the laparoscope and not the camera.

The ultimate for the integral unit is the chip placed on the distal end of the endoscope with only the light-carrying fibers and the electrical wires from the chip passing through the laparoscope. This improves image quality and lighting, since there is no loss of light form transmission through the rod lens system of the laparoscope. These systems are lightweight and have excellent bright images, but for the moment they do not have the versatility of an angled end of the instrument. The lack of need for a proximal camera reduces the size and weight of the instruments.

There is one unit that overcomes the problem of angulation in a combined unit of laparoscope and camera by having a four way deflectable tip that is controlled by an electric motor. The only disadvantage with this unit is the length of the radius of arc of the tip of the laparoscope, which requires considerable space within the abdominal cavity to bend the instrument and at the same time see the area in question while using the instruments.

Although some of these cameras are sophisticated and of high quality, it should be remembered that pieces of a system should match one another. There is no merit to a good camera linked to a poor laparoscope, a poor light source, or a poor monitor. The smaller the endoscopes the greater the problems with light transmission, particularly when the viewing field is large.

III. DIGITIZATION OF THE VIDEO IMAGE

There is a unit that can be purchased that converts the analog signal fed from the current CCD cameras into a digital signal for display on the standard video monitor. The picture quality and image resolution of the resultant image are excellent, with the fine detail of the picture being extremely clear. It is even said that there is some depth perception. The image is not three-dimensional but a standard two-dimensional image; the clearer image gives the feeling of three-dimensionality because there is a marked improvement in the standard two-dimensional depth cues.

It must be remembered that the magnified image is not a true digital image, since the original image from the CCD camera is in fact analog. This is an interim technology until the digital video chips are developed completely and are on the market at a reasonable cost. When the whole image is digital, from the chip to the display, it is likely that it will permit good use of an electronic zoom without loss of definition and resolution during magnification.

IV. Video Monitors

The design of the video monitor is based on the cathode ray tube with a phosphorescent screen. The resolution of a video monitor depends on the number of lines on the screen and the cycling rate. The greater the number of lines and the higher the cycling rate, the better is the definition, assuming that a good quality input signal was used. The standard television has 488 lines, and most monitors are in the region of 640 lines. Some monitors are significantly higher at 1040 lines. The average video monitor cycles at 50 Hz, but a better resolution is possible with rates of 75 Hz. Another feature is the size of the monitor. An image will often appear to have poorer resolution on a large monitor than a small monitor with the same number of lines when each monitor is viewed from the same distance. However, this is not an issue when the observer views the screen from the correct distance, which is considered to be four times the width of the screen.

The optimal placement of the video monitor around the operating table, to provide the surgeon with the best view and the most efficient manual dexterity, is not always considered when positioning all the other equipment that is required to perform a laparoscopic procedure. The positioning of other equipment placement should not take preference around the table. More attention should be given to this problem of the optimal position for a monitor. The ideal position for optimal manual dexterity is with the surgeon looking in the line of his/her hands and instruments, in other words, looking in the same direction as he/she would if performing the same task under direct vision. Unfortunately, since this is not possible because of the size and bulk of current video monitors, the next best position must be used. This is considered to be in the line of the hands and instruments but a little below eye level so that the surgeon is looking down. At the same time the ideal distance of the monitor from the surgeon must be considered, and this is thought to be four times the screen width. Too often the monitor is placed off to the side of the patient so that the surgeon has to look to the side, causing fatigue, neck discomfort, and reduction of manual dexterity.

V. PICTURE IN PICTURE

There are times during laparoscopy when it is necessary to view more than one set of information of images, usually two images, at the same time, which means using a second screen. For instance, while performing an endoscopic exploration of a common duct, it is necessary to see the area of insertion of the choledochoscope into the cystic duct and at the same time to see what is happening in the common duct. This requires a second camera, which is attached to the choledochoscope. Or when performing laparoscopic ultrasound, it is necessary to not only view the ultrasound images but also to view the area that is being examined through the laparoscope. There are other instances when more than one screen is needed, such as in fluoroscopy. Not only is it difficult looking from screen to screen to view the information, but the area around the operating table becomes crowded. It is often impossible to place yet another monitor in a position that permits good visualization around the crowded operating table. This can be overcome by using a picture-in-picture editor that permits two images to be displayed on the same monitor at the same time. The size and position of the second picture can be varied, and placed in any position on the monitor. The surgeon is usually working off one image and monitoring the other images. The two images can be changed to make either image the dominant image, depending on for which image more detail is required. Not only does it make it easier to look at one video monitor, but it reduces the amount of equipment needed around an already crowded operating table.

There are other instances when more than one screen is needed during laparoscopy. For instance, when fluoroscopy is being used to aid in common duct exploration with baskets for radiological extraction of common duct stones without the aid of choledochoscopy.

This picture in picture technology can be incorporated into a head-mounted display unit so that the operating surgeon can be fed a variety of important visual information to which he/she may need to refer during a laparoscopic operation. This information may be X rays of transhepatic studies or ERCP films, CT scans, or MRI scans. It avoids the surgeon's having to leave the operating field to walk over to an X-ray screen to view films. The X rays can be constantly referred to by having the relevant X ray miniaturized in the corner of the screen.

Unfortunately, at the present time the picture control is managed by a nurse or technician who is not scrubbed; eventually it may be possible to control the equipment from the sterile field, either with controls in a sterile sheath, voice activation, or by retinal reflex in a head-mounted display.

VI. THREE-DIMENSIONAL VIDEO IMAGING

The big disadvantage of current endoscopic imaging is the two-dimensionality of the image; the image is flat and without depth perception. The two-dimensional camera further requires the use of two-dimensional depth cues to compensate for the lack of depth perception, and these cues are less useful the more complicated the

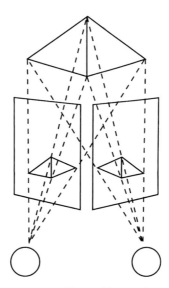

FIGURE 3.1. Normal binocular vision.

task (see Figs. 3.1 and 3.2). There are several three-dimensional laparoscopic units on the market. Although several disadvantages
still need to be ironed out, laparoscopic images have been shown in
studies to improve task performance by 25%. The laparoscope is
not hard to use in the clinical setting, so the learning curve is very
short. Over the next few years three-dimensional imaging will im-

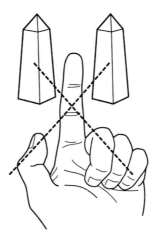

FIGURE 3.2. Demonstration of disparity.

prove and is likely to become the standard for laparoscopic visualization (see Fig. 3.3).

The most common format for 3-D laparoscopic systems is a two-channel laparoscope or a single-channel laparoscope with stereoscopic lens at either end of the instrument such that two stereoscopic images, exhibiting parallax and stereopsis, are delivered to the proximal end of the laparoscope. Two cameras are attached to the proximal end of the laparoscope that individually record each image, the right camera for the right-sided image and the left camera for the left image. The images from each camera are alternately cycled onto a video monitor at 120 Hz and, when the resultant images is viewed, through either active polarized shutter glasses or passive circular polarized glasses. At least one system digitizes and computerizes the image signals prior to display on the monitor.

The images are cycled onto a monitor at 120 Hz, either interlaced or full frame, and observed through active shutter glasses or passive circular polarized glasses. A crystal emitter mounted on the top of the monitor and cycling at 120 Hz in time with the right and left camera signals, controls the active shutter glasses so that the right eye only sees the right eye image and the left eye only sees the

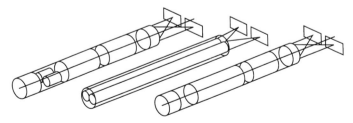

FIGURE 3.3. Three schematic drawing of different 3-D laparoscopic camera designs:
- The top design has a common optical channel with binocular lenses on the distal end of the laparoscope which focus the images on two separate cameras.
- The middle design has two separate optical channels that focuses the images on two separate cameras.
- The lower design has a common optical channel that focuses the images on two separate cameras.

left eye image. The passive glasses system consists of an active polarizing screen cycling at 120 Hz and mounted on the front of the
monitor. This active screen polarizes the right eye image in a right
circular manner and the left eye image in a left circular manner so
that, when viewed through glasses that have passive lenses with the
right eye lens polarized in a right circular manner and the left eye
lens in a left circular manner, only the respective images are seen as
if in three dimensions. Cycling the right and left eye images at 120
HZ is too fast for the brain to see as separate images and as a result
the brain builds up a three-dimensional image (see Figs. 3.4 and 3.5).

The active shutter glasses have some disadvantages: They are
heavy because of the electronics and the batteries in the sides of the
glasses, there is a flickering that comes from the lights in the operating room that cycle at a different rate, the glasses are fragile and expensive. On the other hand, the passive glasses are cheap and light,
and there is no interference from the lights in the operating room.
There is an element of eye strain and fatigue during a long procedure with the active glasses system that is not present with the passive glasses.

The major disadvantage of three-dimensional imaging is the
darkness of the image caused by the small binocular optical channels in the laparoscope, which limit the amount of light transfer to
each CCD camera; the cycling rate of 120 Hz limits the time of presentation of each image on the monitor for half the normal time be-

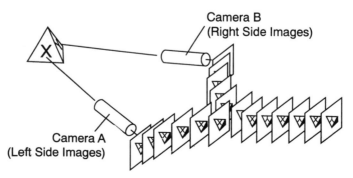

FIGURE 3.4. A schematic demonstration of the cycling of the images
from each camera.

What your eyes see

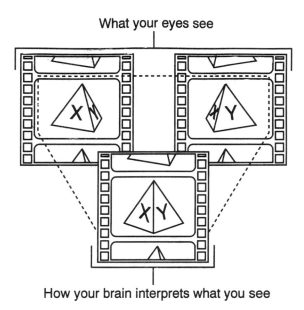

How your brain interprets what you see

FIGURE 3.5. A schematic demonstration of the interpretation of the right and left camera images built into a three dimensional image by the brain.

cause of the competition of the right and left eye images for image projection. The image on the monitor also is dark because of the darkness of the polarized lenses of the glasses.

In some systems the rapid cycling and the slow refresh rate of the monitor has resulted in the need to cycle in an interlacing manner, where half of the monitor lines are used by the right eye image and the other half are used by the left eye image. Some systems have the ability to cycle full frame, using all the lines of the monitor. This results in a brighter image.

Some companies have compensated for this darkness by using high-intensity light sources. One company has compensated for the darkness by doing away with the rod lens optics and mounting two CCD chips on the distal end of the laparoscopes. This design gives the brightest image of any of the 3-D laparoscopic systems.

We have performed experiments to compare 2-D and 3-D imaging systems and found that simple one-handed manipulations in a trainer were as fast in 2-D as in 3-D imaging. However, for more complicated two-handed manipulations in a trainer, the exercises were performed 25% faster in 3-D than in 2-D.[2]

These systems are expensive and cannot be put together piecemeal by purchasing the components separately. The equipment consists of specific and dedicated instruments that must be purchased as one integral unit. One company has reduced the cost issue by designing a 3-D system that integrates with components of an existing 2-D system that is already in the operating room. Their system uses an existing 2-D laparoscope, light source, and 2-D CCD camera. A coupler is provided that fits between the laparoscope and the camera; the coupler's shutter moves from side to side at 120 Hz, and delivers to the single camera a binocular image generated alternately, at 120 Hz, so that each side of the single-channel laparoscope is observed. The signals from the camera are delivered to a signal-processing unit that cycles the right and the left eye images to the monitor at 120 Hz in a full frame manner. This system has true measurable depth perception with a bright image and excellent resolution.

The three-dimensional laparoscopes could be improved by introducing head-mounted displays. Such a system would do away with the need to cycle the images, since presently the right eye cannot see the left eye screen, and the left eye cannot see the right eye screen. Then the right eye image could be continuously delivered to the right eye screen and the left eye image continuously delivered to the left eye screen. The lack of cycling and the lack of polarizing glasses would result in brighter images.

VII. EMERGING VISUALIZATION TECHNOLOGY

VIDEO SCREENS OF THE FUTURE

Over the next few years the video display techniques are going to move away from the present video monitors in the direction of new screen technology that will enhance the quality of the image and the method of viewing it. Some of these techniques will include the following themes, or variations on them depending on the direction of their development.

HEAD-MOUNTED DISPLAYS

The large video monitors used during a laparoscopic operation are not ideal for these procedures because they are large, bulky, and hard to place in a good position where they can be easily and comfortably seen by the surgeon, his assistants, and the nursing staff. The use of two monitors makes it easier for the operating team but increases the amount of equipment around the operating table. It is important in a laparoscopic procedure to optimize the manual dexterity of the surgeon, and to achieve this, the position of the monitor is critical. It needs to be placed at eye level in the same horizontal line as the line of the surgeon's instruments. However, because of the size of these monitors, the surgeon often ends up looking to one side or the other. There is also a suggestion that dexterity is improved if the monitor is placed exactly in line with the axis of the instruments instead of horizontally in line with the instruments at the eye level of the surgeon. This could be achieved by the surgeon's wearing a head-mounted display unit that contains two small liquid crystal display screens, one placed in front of each eye. In this way the surgeon can drop his head on the axis of the instruments in a more relaxed position, and at the same time the head of an assistant does not get in the way of the monitor. Another advantage is the lack of distraction from activities in the operating room taking place in the vicinity of a standard monitor.

This ideal has not yet been completely reached. Currently the several disadvantages of existing systems are slowly being corrected as improvements develop. The main problem is that the definition on the LCD screen has remained poor, since the pixel density of most screens is in the range of 180,000 pixels. This low pixel density results in a lot of grain on the screen that interferes with the definition of the image. Screens are constantly being improved, and the pixel density of the screens currently under development are in the 500,000 pixel density range. That range gives a picture of the same quality as the television. The pixel density in the near future will be above this level, enabling excellent quality images. Other problems with the current generation of head-mounted displays are the weight of the equipment and its instability on the head. The equipment needs to be lighter and the techniques for stabilizing it on the head need to be improved. One of the problems is the need to have the screens some distance in front of the surgeon so that the instruments can be viewed by looking down at them and the patient's abdomen, which means that the screens must project some distance in front of the surgeon, and this creates a leveraging effect on the head band which contributes to the instability.

Head-mounted displays have great potential for three-dimensional imaging, since the right and the left eye images do not have to be alternately cycled onto one screen with the use of shutter glasses or passive circular polarized glasses permitting only the correct eye to see the correct eye image. The right eye image can be continuously projected on to the right LCD screen, and the left eye image can be continuously projected onto the left eye screen. The image is brighter because the lack of cycling permits each image to be projected on the respective screens for twice the length of time and the operator does not have to wear darkened polarizing glasses. Perfection of the head-mounted display technique will increase the use of three-dimensional imaging in laparoscopic operations.

SMALL HAND-HELD LCD SCREENS

A small "all in one" camera and LCD screen has just come onto the market. The unit is compact, comprising a single CCD chip video camera attached to a small LCD screen by a ball joint to enable the position of the screen to be moved around into the best position for viewing. It can be easily attached to any of the standard rigid or flexible endoscopic instruments. The screens come in two sizes, 4 and 6 cm wide, and they have a pixel density of 180,000 pixels. This gives a picture with a resolution on these small screens that is poor but is good enough for office procedures or a quick diagnostic laparoscopy. As the resolution of the LCD screens improves with higher pixel density, and cameras with three CCD chips are developed, these units may have a wide application.

FLAT SCREEN TECHNOLOGY

The nature of monitors is changing, the old cathode ray tube with its bulk and large size is being replaced by flat screens that are thin and light. This technology at the moment is expensive, but with further development and a fall in price, these monitors may play an important part in laparoscopy. With thin screens it will be possible to swing them over the table and place them over the chest of the patient in front of the anesthesiologist or in any other position that is the direct line of the operating surgeon. The position of directly in front of the surgeon in the line of his hands is the optimal position for maximal dexterity.

THREE-DIMENSIONAL GLASSES-FREE SCREENS

There is are effort under way to produce a video monitor on which a three-dimensional image can be displayed with true measurable depth perception, excellent resolution, and true color display but viewed without the need to wear shuttered or passive polarized glasses. One of the prototype models is a unique LCD screen with backlight technology called parallax illumination. The current screen, which is approximately 10×12 in., consists of an LCD screen with an illuminating plate located behind the LCD screen that generates a set of very thin, very bright, uniformly spaced vertical lines. These lines are spaced with respect to the pixel columns and the head of the observer when he/she is situated 30 in. in front of the screen; the observer's left eye sees all the odd columns of the LCD screen while the right eye all the even pixel columns of the LCD screen. The three-dimensional video camera cycles the right and left eye images at 120 Hz so that the right eye image is displaced on the even pixel columns and the left eye image on the odd pixel columns. The observer can move his/her head to a limited degree, since there is a built-in head-tracking system that follows the observer's head movements, activating a dynamic parallax illuminating system that alters the bright lines of the backlight mechanism thereby causing the three-dimensional image projection to follow the observer's eyes. This dynamic parallax system allows the three-dimensional image to follow the observer's eyes, but there is a slight flicker as the observer moves his/her head. Since the screens are LCD screens, they are thin and lightweight, and they can be individualized so that each member of the operation team views his own screen.

At the moment the pixel density of the LCD screen is low at 180,000 and 310,000 pixels, which are densities that produce a poor-quality image that is very grainy and lacking acceptable resolution. This deficiency in resolution will improve as the pixel density of the screens is raised. Densities of 500,000 pixels provides the same resolution as a television screen but higher pixel densities are required to match the resolution of the currently available video monitors. These levels of pixel density on LCD screens will be achieved in the next few years. Until such pixel densities are available, the resolution will not be good enough for the performance of safe and accurate laparoscopic procedures. Nevertheless, a major drawback of the screens remains in the need to keep the head in a relatively small focal area to adequately see the screen without distortion, something that is extremely hard to do when performing a laparoscopic procedure.

VISTRAL FRAMES

Vistral frame imaging is a simple technique that significantly sharpens the image and is likely to come into common use. The technology involves the placing of a broad frame a little in front of the screen to enhance the image and give the image a three-dimensional impression. While there is no true measurable depth perception, the vistral frame does reduce the flat image effect of the standard monitor.

SUSPENDED SCREENS

A still developing technology for image display is that of the suspended image. Using this technology the monitor would be replaced by a technique of suspending the image over the patient's abdomen so that the image is in the line of the operator's hands. This would remove the bulk of equipment, provide a high-quality image exactly where it is needed, right over the patient's body. The fact that the image is now in the same line as the surgeon's hands will improve the dexterity of the surgeon and remove the problem of looking off to the side at a monitor, it will produce more of the feeling of three-dimensional imaging.

Both techniques are likely to play an important part in two-dimensional imaging in the future.

VIRTUAL RETINAL DISPLAY

There is an emerging technology of Virtual Retinal Display (VRD) (MicroVision, Inc., Seattle, WA) that may have great potential for video endoscopic surgery and, as result, may solve some of the major objections to other visualization technologies. The current video monitor is bulky, however, and difficult to place around the operating table so that the surgeon and the assistants can have a comfortable, unobstructed view free from surrounding distractions of the room. Head-mounted displays are on the horizon, but they have potential drawbacks. The units are likely to be somewhat heavy and awkward to wear, the pixel density of the screens is low (which results in a poor quality image); and the currently projected units will make it difficult to view the abdominal wall and trocars impeding the view of the instruments.

Virtual Retinal Display does not create an image that is external to the eye but focuses a fine beam of light projected in raster patterns onto the retina. The video/graphic source emits a fine beam of light of extremely low power (400 nw), which is rapidly scanned across the retina by a horizontal scanner and by a vertical scanner that controls movement of the beam to the next line of pixels to be scanned. The scanning is so rapid that the viewer sees a stable and continuous image that fills the whole eye and has none of the limitations of a video screen. Currently, the image has a VGA resolution of 640 by 480 pixels; however, this pixel density will soon increase. The unit will be small and lightweight, with a video/graphic source mounted on the side of the head that focuses the beam of light onto a small mirror suspended in front of the eye which reflects the image onto the retina. A three-dimensional image can be generated with a video/graphic source mounted on each side of the head, with the image from the stereoscopic laparoscopic cameras focused onto the respective retinas. The small size of the units will make the weight of the head units light and therefore both easier to wear and more stable on the head than head-mounted display units. It will also be easier to visualize the abdomen, using either "see-through" technology or having a sterile control unit to turn one or both units off to permit the surgeon to see the room and the abdomen.

The ultimate goal is to provide an image that occupies the whole retina so that the surgeon experiences a feeling of total immersion without any distraction within the room and at the same time is in a comfortable position while viewing the projected image.

VIII. OTHER IMAGING EQUIPMENT

HIGH-DEFINITION TELEVISION (HDTV)

High-definition television has introduced a new format for the transmission of televised images. This new format has a new screen size with an aspect ratio of 16:9, making it much broader than the current monitors with an aspect ratio of 4:3. The capability of image reproduction is much higher with five to six times more detail. The result is a very sharp image with sharper details and more peripheral vision. The definition is so good that it is almost life-like, and there appears to be depth to the images despite the two-dimensional imaging.

The equipment for the moment is extremely heavy and bulky as well as extremely expensive. The units are selling for between $100,000 and $200,000. The equipment is too big and heavy to be brought into the operative field, and it must be hung from the ceiling and connected to the endoscope with a articulating arm with mirrors. While HDTV has been used to perform laparoscopic procedures, it is too expensive and bulky to be practical as yet. The sharp definition of the picture by far surpasses the definition on even the best imaging equipment of today. With the further development of the technology combined with its introduction into commercial broadcasting, the equipment will be miniaturized and the cost will come down more reasonable levels. At that time it may become a practical imaging medium for laparoscopic procedures.

This technology has been used for three-dimensional HDTV projection, but it is a very complicated, bulky, and expensive technology at the moment. The two stereoscopic images from the laparoscope are projected through an articulated arm with mirrors attached to two HDTV cameras. The images are then cycled and projected as three dimensional on an HDTV monitor viewed through polarizing glasses to direct the correct image to the correct eye. Currently the cost of three-dimensional HDTV equipment is extremely high.

LAPAROSCOPIC ULTRASOUND

Ultrasound is becoming increasingly important in body imaging
because it is easy to use, lacks radiation, and is safe for the patient.
Visual imaging is the mainstay of laparoscopy. However, for maximal assessment of the peritoneal cavity, visual imaging must be
combined with other methods of visualization, of which the most
promising is ultrasound, since it combines visualization of the
depths of the abdominal cavity which cannot be accessed by palpa-
tion as is customary in an open operation. Unfortunately, the gray-
scale image of ultrasonography is not as easy for the surgeon to interpret as X rays or CT scans, and it requires formal training. In
abdominal surgery, ultrasonography is used both transcutaneously
and laparoscopically. The different depth of ultrasound penetration
required with each of these techniques determines the frequency of
the probe to be used. The greater the depth of penetration of trans-
cutaneous ultrasonography requires a lower frequency probe in the
range of 2.5 MHz, whereas the smaller depth of penetration required by laparoscopic ultrasound because of direct contact of organs permits the use of higher frequencies of 7.5 MHz. The resolution of the resultant image increases, the higher the frequency of the
probe. Other factors that improve the resolution of the laparoscopic
ultrasound image are, for example, the lack of interference of the
rib cage in the upper abdomen and the interference of the abdominal wall giving rise to such artifacts as the "ring down effect" produced by distortion and reflection of the sound waves by the fascial
plains of the abdominal wall.

The ultrasound probe is made up of a piezoelectric transmitter
crystal that produces sound waves when deformed by an electrical
current and a receiving piezoelectric crystal that turns the reflected
sound waves into an electric current that is then displayed on an
oscilloscope. These piezoelectric crystals are arranged in one of two
patterns on the tips of the ultrasound probe, either as a sector scan
or a linear array probe. In a sector scan probe the crystals are on the
tip of the probe and are arranged to provide a wedge- or pie-

shaped image from the probe, whereas in a linear array probe the crystals are arranged along the side of the end of the probe and give a linear, rectangular side view. It is individual preference that tends to dictate which type of probe is used. If a linear array probe is used laparoscopically, then the probe is arranged to articulate so that satisfactory tissue contact can be achieved. The laparoscopic probes are 10 mm in diameter and are either linear array or sector scan probes. Because of the problem of obtaining good tissue contact with the linear array probes from a fixed access port, these probes are steerable, either two-way or four-way steerable. With the small contact area of the sector scan probe, there is no need for a steerable probe. The most convenient way to display the image during laparoscopic ultrasound is using a picture-in-picture arrangement so that the surgeon can see the placement of the probe as well as the ultrasound image without having to keep looking between two screens. Some ultrasound probes have Doppler ultrasound incorporated into the probe, which permits the distinguishing of blood vessels or other fluid-filled structures.

John et al. find a high accuracy in predicting unresectability for carcinoma of the head of the pancreas and periampullary region when assessing these patients with diagnostic laparoscopy combined with laparoscopic ultrasound prior to laparotomy for attempted resection.[3]

FUTURE DEVELOPMENTS IN LAPAROSCOPIC ULTRASOUND

There is significant room for improvement in the method of displaying the resultant ultrasonographic image. Currently several attempts are made to provide more information and make the image more user friendly. One reflects an early interest in displaying the ultrasonographic image as a three-dimensional image. The three-dimensionality is generated by rotating the probe in two planes at the same time, side to side and back and forth. The technology is in an early stage of development but shows promise.

There is also investigational work under way to display the ultrasound image in a more user-friendly way allowing software manipulation of the data so that the image can be reconstructed as in a CAT scan. This work is still at an early stage, and the images currently look like a first-generation CAT scan. However, the images are much easier for the surgeon to interpret than the gray-scale images in use today. One of the disadvantages at the moment is that the images are not in real time. The software program requires a fast computer to handle the image construction with a current delay of several minutes. Once this aspect of image creation has been overcome, and the images become real time, the technology will markedly enhance its use laparoscopically in conjunction with the endoscopic view of the peritoneal cavity.

IX. CONCLUSION

The current state of laparoscopic visualization by three-chip analog CCD cameras gives a bright, sharp image with highly acceptable definition and color resolution. The analog signal is now being digitized for a clearer definition of the image. These cameras provide a two-dimensional image with no depth perception. The two-dimensional depth cues have to be used to find the relationships of structures to one another. Three-dimensional imaging is currently being used and gives good depth perception, but the images tend to be dark. The technology is now definitely at a stage where it can be used to great effect in laparoscopic procedures, but needs further development. In the near future the video monitor as we know it today will be replaced by more sophisticated imaging displays that can give sharp definition with less bulky equipment.

Visual examination of the abdominal cavity will be supplemented by ultrasound imaging which is likely to become three dimensional, making it easier for the surgeon to interpret the image and aiding the surgeon in his dissection and understanding of the deeper tissues of the intraabdominal viscera.

REFERENCES

1. Kelling G: Uber Oesophagoskopie, Gastroskopie und Keoliskopie. Read before the 73rd Versamm. Deutch. Naturforscher Und Artze, Hamburg. September 23, 1901. Munchen Med Wchnscher. 1092 Jan: 21.

2. Birkett DH, Josephs LG, Estes-McDonald J: A new 3-D laparoscope in gastrointestinal surgery. *Surg Endosc* (1994) 8:1445–1451.

3. John TG, Greig JD, Crosbie JL, Miles WF, Garden OJ: Carcinoma of the head of the pancreatic head and periampullary region. Tumor staging with laparoscopy and laparoscopic ultrasonography. *Ann Surg* (1995) 221:156–164.

Microelectromechanical Systems (MEMS)

Kaigham J. Gabriel, Ph.D

I. Introduction

As computers increasingly leave fixed locations and appear in the pockets and palms of users, they are getting closer to the physical world, creating new opportunities for perceiving and controlling the physical environment. To exploit these opportunities, computers will need to *sense* and *act* as well as *compute*. Filling this need is the driving force for the development of microelectromechanical systems (MEMS).

Using the fabrication techniques and materials of microelectronics as a basis, MEMS processes construct both *mechanical* and electrical components. Mechanical components in MEMS, like transistors in microelectronics, have dimensions that are measured in microns and numbers measured from a few to millions. MEMS is not about any one single application or device, nor is it defined by a single fabrication process or limited to a few materials. More than anything else, MEMS is a fabrication approach that conveys the

Cybersurgery: Advanced Technologies for Surgical Practice,
Edited by Richard M. Satava, M.D.
ISBN 0-471-15874-7   Copyright © 1998 by Wiley-Liss, Inc.

advantages of miniaturization, multiple components and micro-electronics to the design and construction of integrated *electro-mechanical* systems.

MEMS devices are and will be used widely, with applications ranging from automobiles and fighter aircraft to surgical tools and biomedical implants. While MEMS devices will be a relatively small fraction of the cost, size and weight of these systems, MEMS will be critical to their operation, reliability and affordability. MEMS devices, and the smart products they enable, will increasingly be the performance differentiator for both commercial and defense systems.

This chapter presents an overview of MEMS technology and identifies the key elements and advantages for a variety of micro-machining techniques.

II. CHARACTERISTICS OF MEMS FABRICATION TECHNOLOGIES

Regardless of the specific type of micromachining fabrication process used, all MEMS fabrication approaches share certain key characteristics: *miniaturization, multiplicity,* and *microelectronics.*

Miniaturization is an important but not the sole characteristic of MEMS. There are many advantages to the performance of electro-mechanical devices and systems that come from miniaturization. Structures that are relatively small and light lead to devices that have relatively high resonant frequencies. These high resonant frequencies in turn mean higher operating frequencies and band-widths for sensors and actuators. Thermal time constants, the rate at which structures absorb and release heat, are shorter for smaller, less massive structures. But miniaturization is not the principal driving force for MEMS that it is for microelectronics. Because MEMS devices are by definition interacting with some aspect of the physical world (e.g., pressure, inertia, fluid flows, light), there is a size below which further miniaturization is *detrimental* to device and system operation. For example, reducing the size (and consequently the mass) of an accelerometer makes it harder to detect low-g accelerations. This minimum size is different for different applications, but for most MEMS applications, the size limits are a factor of 3 to 5 larger than the smallest microelectronic device features.

As important as miniaturization, *multiplicity* or the batch fabrication inherent in photolithographic-based MEMS processing, provides two important advantages to electromechanical devices and systems. Multiplicity makes it possible to fabricate 10,000 or a million components as easily, quickly, and at the same time as one component. This advantage of MEMS fabrication is critical for reducing the unit cost of devices, and the semiconductor industry has proved the benefits of such economies of scale. The second, equally important advantage enabled by multiplicity is the additional flexibility in the design of massively-parallel, interconnected electromechanical systems.

Rather than designing components, the emphasis can shift to designing the pattern and form of interconnections (interactions or coordinated action) among thousands or millions of components. This approach to design has been standard operating procedure in microelectronic systems design for nearly three decades. When integrated circuit engineers design and lay out a new circuit, they don't design new components, but instead design the pattern of interconnections among millions of relatively simple and identical components. The diversity and complexity of function in integrated circuits is a direct result of the diversity and complexity of the interconnections, and it is the differences in the interconnections that differentiate a microprocessor from a memory. The multiplicity characteristic of MEMS has already been exploited in the development and recent demonstration of a digital micromirror display. In an array about the size of two standard postage stamps, over a million mirrors, each the size of a red blood cell, collectively generate a complete, high-resolution video image. Trying to build and operate such a display using conventional methods of mechanical component manufacturing and assembly would be nearly impossible and certainly not affordable.

Finally, neither the miniaturization nor the multiplicity characteristics of MEMS could be fully exploited were it not for the *microelectronics* that is merged with the electromechanical components. Whether the electronics processing and micromachining steps are interleaved, the electronics processing precedes the micromachining steps, or the microelectronics processing and the micromachining are done separately and later flip-chip or wire-bonded does not matter. The integrated microelectronics provides the intelligence to MEMS and allows the closed-loop feedback systems, localized signal conditioning, and the control of massively-parallel actuator arrays. Furthermore the considerable and historic investments in microelectronics materials, processing, and expertise will accelerate not only the development of MEMS devices but will also accelerate the acceptance of MEMS devices by systems designers and integrators.

III. FABRICATION METHODS AND MATERIALS

Common processing techniques that are used to sculpt mechanical structures include bulk micromachining, wafer-to-wafer bonding, surface micromachining, and high-aspect ratio micromachining. While the objective of all these techniques is the fabrication of integrated mechanical and electrical structures, some techniques are best suited for MEMS with robust mechanical parts and structure, some for high-precision components, and others for high levels of integrated electrical-mechanical components.

Bulk micromachining is the term applied to a variety of etching procedures that selectively remove material, typically with a chemical etchant whose etching properties are dependent on the crystallographic structure of the bulk material. By using appropriate material coatings and patterning steps to mask the surface of the material (most commonly silicon wafers of the same type used in microelectronics fabrication, but quartz wafers are also used), selective areas of the wafer surface can be exposed to the micromachining etchants. The shape of the etched cavities and etch rates are typically determined by the crystalline structure of the wafer material and the particular etching reaction (a type of etching termed *anisotropic etching*). Additional variations in the type of features and structures are possible by selective and patterned doping (the injection of other atoms, e.g., boron, up to 20 µm into the pure-silicon surface) of the wafer. Doping inhibits the action of the crystalline etches and thus can leave behind free-form structures following a bulk, anisotropic etching of material. Figure 4.1 is an illustration of an example component with a composite of all common features and mechanical structures that can be etched in single-crystal silicon using bulk micromachining. The features and structures range

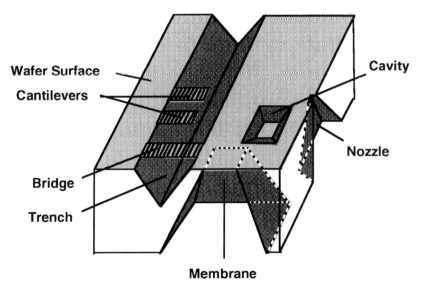

FIGURE 4.1. An arbitrary component with a composite of all common features and mechanical structures that can be etched in a piece of single-crystal silicon using bulk micromachining. Note that all etched walls are at the same angle as defined by the crystal orientation of the silicon (adapted from Mechanical Engineering [3]).

from pyramidal pits and V-groove trenches to membranes and cantilevered beams. The cantilevered beam (the "diving board") and doubly supported beam (the bridge) suspended above the etched V-groove in Figure 4.1 would have been defined by rectangular doping patterns (corresponding to the beam geometries) prior to the etch of the V-groove. Bulk micromachining is an extensively used commercial process, particularly in the production of pressure sensors, accelerometers, and flow regulators.

Wafer-to-wafer bonding is a strategy commonly employed to get around the restrictions in the type of structures that can be fabricated using bulk micromachining. Since anisotropic etching, by definition, only *removes* material, bonding of wafers allows for the *addition* of material to the bulk micromachining repertoire. Wafer-to-wafer bonding is the bonding (under pressure or a combination of pressure and a high voltage across the wafer) of two or more micromachined wafers to construct MEMS. Constituent wafers can be bulk micromachined wafers, wafers with prefabricated electronics, or wafers micromachined by other techniques. In many cases the bonded wafers are silicon-to-silicon, but silicon-to-quartz and silicon-to-pyrex bonds are also common. Wafer-to-wafer bonding is a versatile fabrication technique suitable for processing whole wafers at a time (a wafer-scale technique that maintains the advantages of batch fabricated processes) and yields high-quality interfaces and bonds. Heavy commercial use of wafer-to-wafer bonding is made in the production of pressure sensors and integrated fluidic systems (flow valves and regulators, ink-jet nozzles, pumps, chemical sensors, and miniature analytical instruments).

Despite the usefulness of bulk micromachining and wafer-to-wafer bonding (and their continuing commercial importance), these micromachining techniques are limiting in the type of features that can be sculpted. Bulk micromachined structures and features are defined by the internal crystalline structure of the material. Fabricating multiple, interconnected electromechanical parts of free-form geometry using bulk micromachining is often difficult or impossible. While wafer-to-wafer bonding gets around some of these limitations, truly free-form geometries and integrated multicomponent (multiple, interconnected, and cofabricated components) electromechanical structures are presently produced by a relatively new micromachining approach that is fundamentally different from bulk micromachining and wafer-to-wafer bonding.

Surface micromachining, like bulk micromachining, also starts with a wafer of material. But unlike bulk micromachining where the wafer itself serves as the stock from which material is removed to define mechanical structures, in surface micromachining the wafer is the substrate—the working surface—on which multiple, alternating layers of structural and sacrificial material are deposited and etched (Fig. 4.2). A typical cycle in a surface micromachining process begins with a deposition of either the sacrificial material (a material that will be completely removed in the final step of the fabrication process) or the structural material (a material from which the functional components of the electromechanical system will be constructed). The layer is then masked with a desired pattern which is typically transferred using a photolithographic process, usually the exposure of a photosensitive material (photoresist) and development (removal) of the exposed photoresist. Next the underlying material not protected by the masking pattern is etched, typically by reactive ion etching (a sort of sand blasting with ions) to transfer the mask pattern to that particular material layer. The deposition-masking-etching cycle is repeated on all the laminated layers of structural and sacrificial materials until the MEMS device structure is complete. The final step in surface micromachining is the release of the structural material from the laminations by etching or removing the underlying and surrounding sacrificial materials.

The most commonly used surface micromachining processes start with silicon wafers of the same grade and type used in microelectronics fabrication and use layers of silicon dioxide as the sacrificial material and layers of polysilicon (a deposited, less crystalline

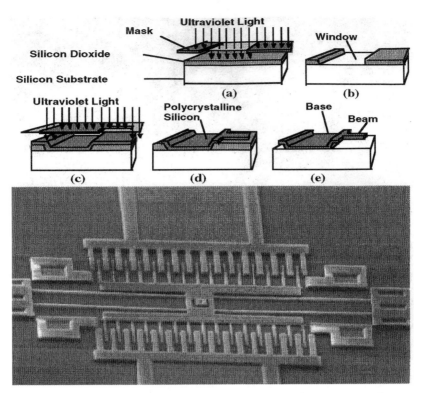

FIGURE 4.2. A single cycle in a common surface micromachining process. The process to build a single cantilever beam begins with the sacrificial material layer (silicon dioxide) being patterned and etched (*a*, *b*). Next the structural material (polysilicon) is deposited over the entire surface. The polysilicon is then patterned and etched in the shape of the cantilever beam and base (*c*, *d*). Finally the polysilicon is released by removing the remaining and underlying silicon dioxide (*e*). A portion of the patterned polysilicon is attached to the substrate forming the base (where the silicon dioxide was removed), and portions are suspended above the substrate and free to move (where the silicon dioxide had remained). The scanning electron microscope picture is a side view of a comb-drive resonator fabricated with such a sequence. Note the two tri-indented square anchors which are the base holding the rest of the central folded beam and comb structures suspended above the substrate.[2]

form of silicon) as the structural material. Other deposited materials such as silicon nitride, polyimides, and aluminum are also extensively used to provide electrically insulating materials, conducting materials, etchant masks, and additional structural materials. All of these materials are extensively available and used in standard microelectronics fabrication.

Because of the laminated structural and sacrificial material layers and the etching of material done by a process that is insensitive to crystalline structure (either because of the etch or because the material itself is noncrystalline), surface micromachining enables the fabrication of free-form, complex and multicomponent integrated electromechanical structures, liberating the MEMS designer to envision and build devices and systems that are impossible to realize with bulk or bonded processes. Surface micromachining also frees the process developer and device designer to choose any material system that has complementary structural and sacrificial materials (structural materials that are unaffected by the etching of the sacrificial material). Examples of other material pairs include metals as structural materials paired with polyimides as sacrificial materials.

It is this freedom to fabricate devices and systems without constraints on materials, geometries, assembly, and interconnections that is the source for the richness and depth of MEMS applications which cut across so many areas. *More than any other factor, it is surface micromachining that has ignited and is at the heart of the current scientific and commercial activity in MEMS.*

IV. MEMS DEVICE EXAMPLES

Two examples of MEMS devices are the ADXL50, manufactured by Analog Devices, Inc., and the Digital Micromirror Device (DMD), a product of Texas Instruments, Inc.

The ADXL50 is a surface-micromachined, complete acceleration measurement system on a single monolithic integrated circuit, with its signal-conditioning circuitry and MEMS structures integrated on the same chip through a customized fabrication process. Figure 4.3 depicts the ADXL50 accelerometer, which has a full-scale measurement range of ±50 g, sensitivity of 19 mV/g, self-test on digital command, and a high shock survival (>2000 g, unpowered).

The ADXL50 has enjoyed widespread market acceptance in the automotive industry, with current and potential uses including airbag, vehicle dynamics and auto security applications.

The DMD is a pixelated, micromechanical spatial light modulator formed monolithically on a silicon substrate using a standard, 5-V, 0.8-μm CMOS process. Each of these 16 μm × 16 μm micromirrors (Fig. 4.4) contributes to an overall projection display featuring 2000 × 1000 pixel resolution (2 million micromirror array, sample in Fig. 4.5).

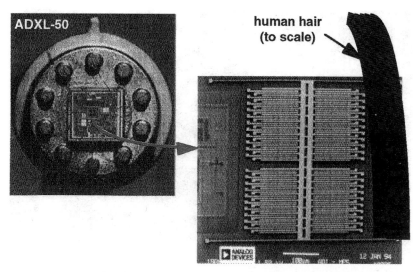

FIGURE 4.3. Surface-micromachined MEMS accelerometer, bonded wafer photograph (*left*), and scanning electron micrograph (SEM, *right*). The ADXL50 has successfully demonstrated high accuracy and linearity through harsh industrial conditions, a necessary trait for use in automotive applications (Analog Devices, Inc.).

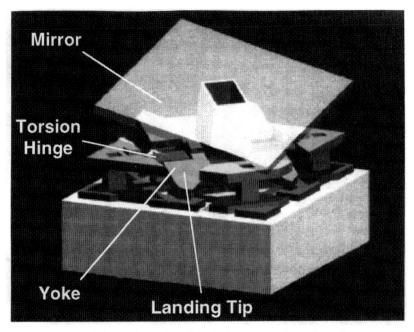

FIGURE 4.4. Illustration of DMD pixel cross section (Texas Instruments, Inc.).

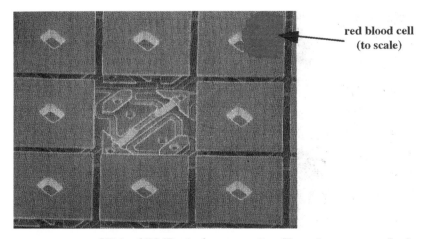

FIGURE 4.5. SEM of DMD pixel cross section (Texas Instruments, Inc.).

V. COMPARISON OF MEMS AND MICROELECTRONICS TECHNOLOGIES

Although MEMS fabrication uses many of the materials and processes of semiconductor fabrication, there are important distinctions between the two technologies. The most significant distinctions between MEMS fabrication and semiconductor fabrication are in the process recipes (the number, sequence and type of deposition, removal and patterning steps used to fabricate devices) and in the end-stages of production (bonding of wafers, freeing of parts designed to move, packaging, and test). The fundamental challenge of using semiconductor processes for MEMS fabrication is not in the type of processes and materials used but more in the way those processes and materials are used (Fig. 4.6).

Surface micromachining, the MEMS fabrication technology that uses the most standard microelectronics fabrication processes and materials, is also the one that uses those processes and materials at their extremes. First, the films typically deposited for MEMS are thicker than the films deposited for microelectronics. Whereas microelectronic films are usually in the range of 100s to 1000s of angstroms, MEMS films are usually in the range of 1000s to tens of thousands of angstroms. Second, as a direct consequence of the thicker films, the material removal steps or etches (typically plasma

---

FIGURE 4.6. The manufacturing process flow for a typical microelectronic integrated circuit and a MEMS device. The first phase of the process includes process specification, device design, and mask layout. This is followed by device fabrication, typically multiple slices of material deposition and patterned removal of material. Finally wafers are probed, partitioned into individual devices, packaged, and tested. Despite distinctions in film thicknesses, etch depths, and the release of mechanical structures, the two technologies use the same equipment and materials in the central deposition-photolithography-etch cycles. The significant distinctions between MEMS and electronics processing arise in the electronic design aids and simulators, and in the sectioning, packaging and testing. Examples of these distinctions are shown in italicized, bold text.

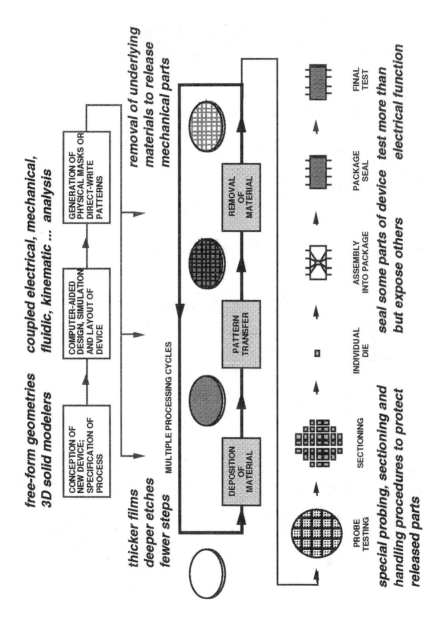

free-form geometries 3D solid modelers

coupled electrical, mechanical, fluidic, kinematic ... analysis

removal of underlying materials to release mechanical parts

| CONCEPTION OF NEW DEVICE; SPECIFICATION OF PROCESS | COMPUTER-AIDED DESIGN, SIMULATION AND LAYOUT OF DEVICE | GENERATION OF PHYSICAL MASKS OR DIRECT-WRITE PATTERNS |

thicker films deeper etches fewer steps

MULTIPLE PROCESSING CYCLES

| DEPOSITION OF MATERIAL | PATTERN TRANSFER | REMOVAL OF MATERIAL |

PROBE TESTING

SECTIONING

INDIVIDUAL DIE

ASSEMBLY INTO PACKAGE

PACKAGE SEAL

FINAL TEST

special probing, sectioning and handling procedures to protect released parts

seal some parts of device but expose others

test more than electrical function

69

and reactive ion etches, often referred to as "dry" etching as opposed to "wet" chemical etching) are necessarily deeper and take longer. Consequently the etch profiles (the shape of the sidewalls in the etched features) become harder to control and maintain to target specification—most often due to undercutting of the etch. Third, the successive buildup of material from multiple depositions, patterning, and etching of material makes the surface of MEMS-processed wafers very non-planar after only a few process cycles. This presents difficulties both for later photolithographic steps (features on prominences in the wafer will be out of focus if features in the depressions are in focus) and later material depositions (thinned areas and even breaks in the surface coverage may occur, particularly at sharp transitions from prominence to depression). Finally, a processing step unique to MEMS is to free or release the parts designed to move (membranes, resonating beams, tiltable mirrors) by removing material underneath portions of these parts. The release of the movable and structural components presents additional considerations for MEMS that are never encountered in microelectronics processing. One important consideration is residual stress inherent in the released films as a result of deposition. If not properly controlled, the stresses will cause the released, mechanical structures to bow and bend, lose their designed shape and orientation, and destroy the functionality of the MEMS devices.

The differences between MEMS and microelectronics process steps illustrate that while MEMS fabrication uses available semiconductor fabrication equipment and processes, the equipment and processes are used in nonstandard ways, often at the extremes of the operating conditions for which they were designed. MEMS will need the development of operating conditions on standard semiconductor equipment suited and optimized to the requirements of MEMS. For other processing steps unique to MEMS, the development of new manufacturing equipment and associated processes will be required.

Only as MEMS are being commercialized and manufacturing realities are identifying production requirements, are we now in a position to begin investments in electronic design aids, MEMS-specific manufacturing equipment, and packaging/interfacing techniques. While advanced MEMS device designs, systems concepts, and fabrication processes will continue to be important, increasingly it is advances in these MEMS-specific manufacturing resources that will pace the developments, commercialization and use of MEMS.

VI. TRENDS IN MEMS TECHNOLOGY

By merging the capabilities of sensors and actuators with information systems, MEMS is extending and increasing the ability to both perceive and control the physical world. To quantitatively measure and track this ability and compare MEMS developments across diverse application areas, a map of electromechanical integration is used as shown in Figure 4.7. The ordinate is a log plot of the number of transistors ranging from one to one billion. Similarly the abscissa is a log plot of the number of mechanical components ranging from one to one billion. To first order, the number of transistors are a measure of information-processing ability, and the number of mechanical components are a measure of perception and control ability.

Plotted on this graph is the region containing the ratios for many historic and current MEMS devices, ratios for some recent advanced MEMS devices, and regions of ratios required for future MEMS technologies and applications.

As can be seen from Figure 4.7, the region containing many current MEMS devices (e.g., pressure sensors, accelerometers, and the flow valve described earlier) is a small area near the lower left of the plot, or the region representing devices with a few mechanical components and a ratio of one to a few transistors per mechanical component. Moving out from this cluster near the origin, regions of higher levels of integrated electronics are generally to the left and top, and regions of greater numbers of mechanical components are

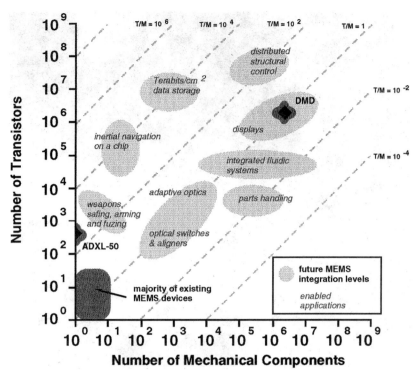

FIGURE 4.7. Log-log plot of number of transistors merged with number of mechanical components for MEMS devices and systems. Contours of equal transistors-to-mechanical-components ratios (T/M) are lines of 45° slope. Lines representing T/M ratios ranging from 10^{-4} to 10^6 are shown for reference. The resulting map represents a quantitative way to measure and track MEMS technology advances across different application areas.[5]

to the right and top. Recent MEMS technology advances have made possible two MEMS devices of higher integration levels and greater number of integrated mechanical components, each developed for completely different applications. These devices are also plotted on this graph. One is the ADXL50, a MEMS accelerometer with approximately 200 transistors to a single mechanical proof mass,[1] and the other is the digital micromirror display (DMD) with approximately six million transistors to two million mechanical micromirrors[4].

In different ways, both of these devices represent significant advances for MEMS technology and MEMS devices capabilities. The ADXL50 has moved up from the current MEMS region onto a higher integrated electronics to mechanics line ($T/M \approx 200$) but has kept the number of mechanical components at one. In contrast, the DMD has stayed on nearly the same processing to perception and control ratio line ($T/M \approx 6$) but has increased the number of both transistors and mechanical components (because of the replicative, identical mirrors and underlying electronics inherent in the structure of the device) by nearly six orders of magnitude.

The higher levels of integrated electronics and the greater number of integrated mechanical components represented by these two MEMS devices quantify the degree of recent MEMS technology advancements. In the context of the entire graph, the two points also illustrate the opportunity in MEMS represented by the regions of processing, perception, and actuation integration yet to be explored. These unexplored regions are not only guides for advances in integration but also to the capabilities that will be enabled at those integration levels. For example, to develop inertial navigation units on a chip will likely require nearly two orders of magnitude increase in both the number of transistors and mechanical components to reach the sensitivity and stability necessary in those devices. In contrast, the development of some fluid pumps or microoptomechanical devices will likely require greater numbers of mechanical components, but at lower levels of integrated electronics than other MEMS applications.

Future MEMS applications will be driven by processes that enable greater functionality through higher levels of electronic-mechanical integration and greater number of mechanical components. These process developments in turn will be paced by investments in the development of new materials, device and systems design, fabrication techniques, packaging/assembly methods, and test and characterization tools.

REFERENCES

1. Core T A, Tsang WK, Sherman SJ: "Fabrication technology for an integrated surface-micromachined sensor." *Solid State Tech* (October 1993).

2. Gabriel, K: "Microelectromechanical systems program: Summary of research activities." Advanced Research Projects Agency, July 1994.

3. Howe RT, et al.: "Micromotor on a chip." *IEEE Spec* (July 1990).

4. Younse JM: "Mirrors on a chip." *IEEE Spec* (November 1993).

5. Gabriel, K: "Engineering microscopic machines." *Sci Am* (September 1995).

VIRTUAL REALITY

Richard M. Satava, M.D., F.A.C.S. and Cdr. Shaun B. Jones, M.D.

There are many different definitions of virtual reality, each depending on the context, point of view, or professional experience of the one making the definition. However, most people will agree with the pragmatic definition of Dr. Tom Furness of the Human Interface Technology Lab at the University of Washington, who describes a virtual environment as "the representation of a computer model or database which can be interactively experienced and manipulated by the participant(s)."[1] There is also the description of the equipment used to create a virtual environment, which provides a sense of being immersed completely within the computer representation; this is often achieved by using a head-mounted display (HMD) and DataGlove™ to separate the user from the real world so that the only physical experience is that which the computer provides. For medicine the computer model usually refers to human anatomy, such as the Visible Human or a patient image from CT or MRI scan, but the model can also include symbolic representations of processes such as inflammation, immune response, or shock or of pure data such as the medical record. From a technical standpoint,

Cybersurgery: Advanced Technologies for Surgical Practice,
Edited by Richard M. Satava, M.D.
ISBN 0-471-15874-7   Copyright © 1998 by Wiley-Liss, Inc.

virtual reality has its roots in the disciplines of 3-D visualization and flight simulation.

Computer and graphic artists first began using 3-D graphic visualization to create video games. In the early 1960s Morton Heilig developed a 3-D video experience called the "Sensorama," which was a motorcycle ride through a metropolitan city (Fig. 5.1). There was a 3-D video monitor, handlebars that controlled the point of view, the sounds of cars, busses, and human activity, and a seat that vibrated and bounced in synchrony with the bumps in the video image. It also included a fan blowing air onto the face to simulate wind and even simulated the smell of garbage to evoke the full sense of being in a overburdened city. Later in the decade, Ivan Sutherland[2] developed the first motion-coupled head-mounted display that placed a pair of miniature video monitors in front of the eyes while a mechanical device tracked head motion. This permitted the view of a computer-generated object (wire-frame cube) to change position as the head moved, giving the appearance of a full 3-D cube.

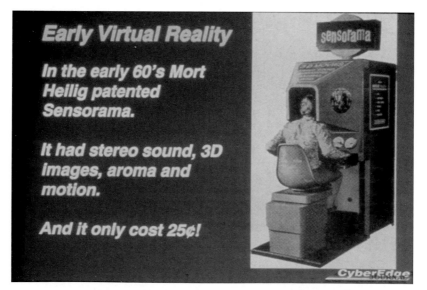

FIGURE 5.1. Morton Heilig's "Sensorama," early 1960s (courtesy of Dr. Joseph Rosen, Dartmouth Medical Center, Lebannon, NH).

It was not until 1985 that NASA developed the familiar current version of HMD[3]. The NASA planetary scientists needed a way to better understand the massive amount of data that was returning from the lunar and Mars probes. Rather than taking the signals from the video cameras on remote planets and converting them into numbers, graphs, and charts, the scientists chose to recreate the visual images and display them on a HMD (Fig. 5.2). In addition the user's ears were covered by a pair of stereophonic speakers; this resulted in a person being completely isolated from the real world and experiencing only the computer-generated "world" that was a visual reconstruction of a planet surface. The addition of the head tracker allowed the person to view the world from any perspective,

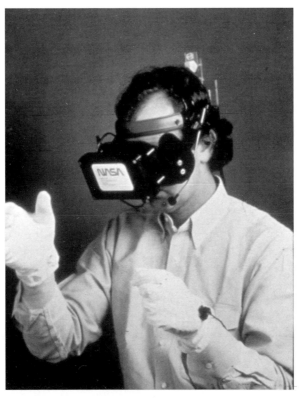

FIGURE 5.2. Dr. Scott Fisher in the early version of NASA head-mounted display with DataGlove™ (courtesy of Dr. Scott Fisher, Palo Alto, CA).

thus being "immersed" in the middle of the data. One must either be sitting on a swivel chair or standing in order to completely turn and move around in the "world." Under these mobile circumstances it is difficult, if not impossible, to be typing on a keyboard or moving a mouse or joystick, so the DataGlove™ was invented. This permitted "grasping" of objects in the virtual world as if they actually existed—using the intuitive motion of handling objects rather than typing commands. Thus a virtual world or environment became an intuitive, immersive way of interacting with a computer, and in some ways the ideal man-machine interface.[4]

The visual fidelity (how realistic it looks) of a virtual environment is dependent on computer power. Today, despite supercomputers, the level of realism is cartoon level; it is almost as if the person were Alice in Wonderland (Fig. 5.3) interacting with cartoonlike characters and objects. They behave and react realistically, but look like cartoons. The more computer power, the more realistic. In 1955 ENIAC (Fig. 5.4) was the first mainframe computer, occupying thousands of square feet, taking numerous engineers to operate, and costing millions of dollars. Today, on a desk top is a computer with thousands of times the power of ENIAC and costing only a thousand dollars. Since computer power is continuing to grow exponentially, it can be expected that in the not too distant future there will be enough power on everyone's desktop that photorealistic images will be commonplace.

The other discipline that gave birth to surgical simulation is flight simulators. In the 1930s pilots like Jimmy Doolittle (Fig. 5.5) were noticing very high accident rates when trying to land at night or in bad weather. By outfitting the plane with instruments (Fig. 5.6), the pilots would take off, zip a canvas over their heads, and attempt to land with only the instruments. Fortunately, just at the same time, Edwin Link began developing a flight simulator (Fig. 5.7). This simulator did not look like a fighter plane because it was a carnival ride that was attached to his father's instruments. (Edwin Link's father was an organ repair man). In spite of the fact that the

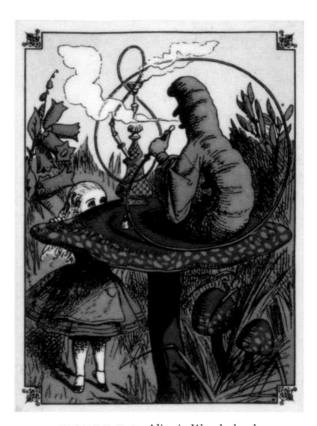

FIGURE 5.3. Alice in Wonderland.

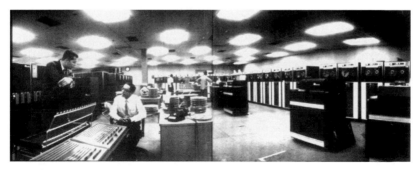

FIGURE 5.4. ENIAC computer, the first mainframe computer (courtesy Dr. Steven Ellis, NASA-Ames, Palo Alto, CA).

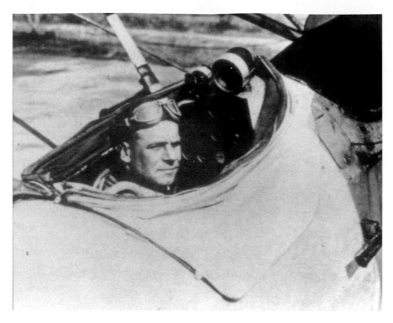

FIGURE 5.5. General Jimmy Doolittle in the 1930s. Notice the canvas that he can zip over his head, once airborne, in order to practice "instruments landings" (courtesy of CAE-Link archives).

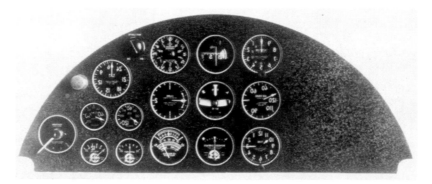

FIGURE 5.6. Very simple instruments used to attempt "instrument landing" (courtesy of CAE-Link archives).

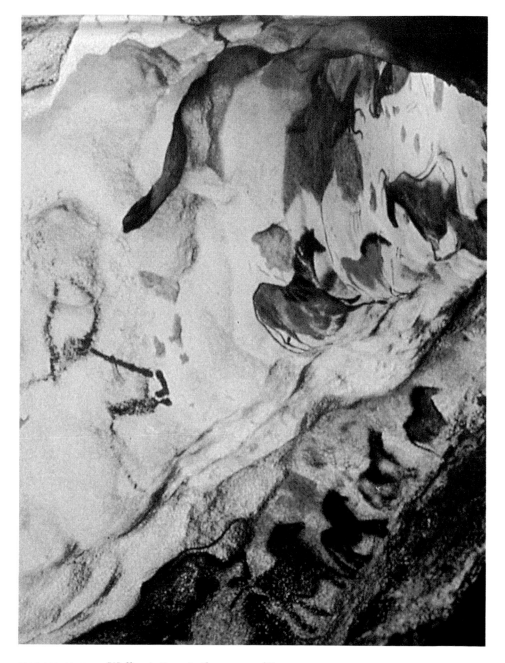

FIGURE 2.1. Wall paintings in the caves of France.

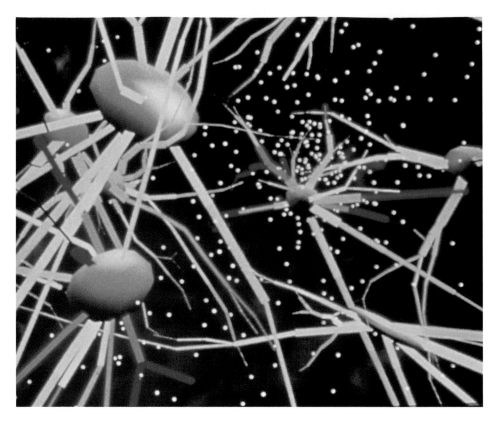

FIGURE 2.6. Graphic representations of brain cells the size of footballs and neurons for display in the CAVE. (Courtesy of Dr. Tom Defanti, University of Illinois, Chicago, IL).

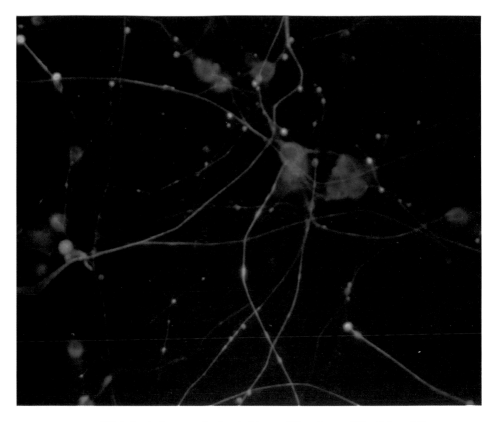

FIGURE 2.7. Histologic image of a brain biopsy (Courtesy of Dr. Brian Athey, University of Michigan, Ann Arbor, MI).

FIGURE 2.9.
Suspended
3-D holographic
image of a
mandible.
(Courtesy of
Jonathan Prince,
Dimensional
Media Associates,
New York City,
NY).

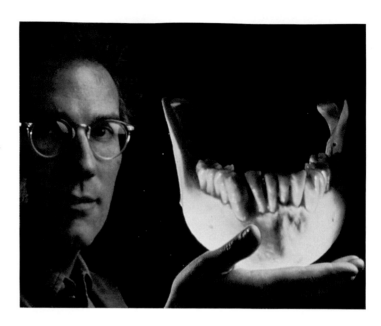

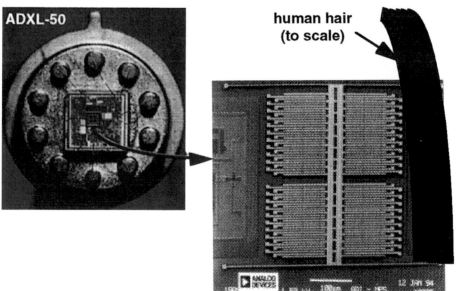

FIGURE 4.3. Surface-micromachined MEMS accelerometer, bonded wafer photograph (left) and scanning electron micrograph (SEM, right). The ADXL50 has successfully demonstrated high accuracy and linearity through harsh industrial conditions, a necessary trait for use in automotive applications (Analog Devices, Inc.).

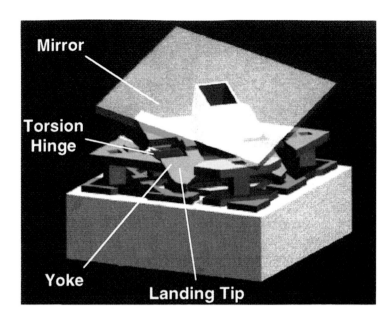

FIGURE 4.4.
Illustration of
DMD pixel
cross-section
(Texas Instruments,
Inc.).

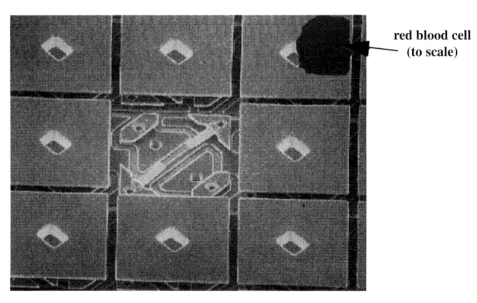

red blood cell
(to scale)

FIGURE 4.5. SEMS of DMD pixel cross-section (Texas
Instruments, Inc.).

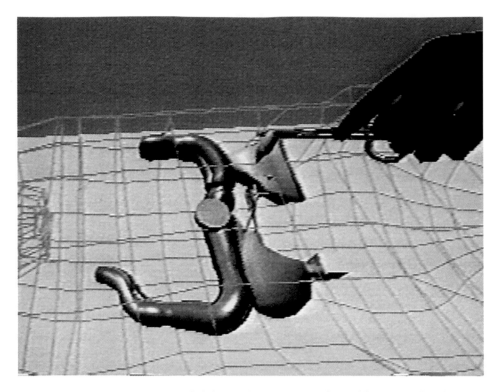

FIGURE 5.10. Early version of abdominal surgery simulator. (Courtesy of author).

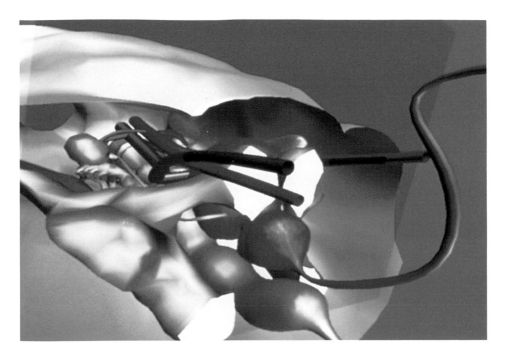

FIGURE 5.11. Second generation surgical simulator, with tissue properties (Courtesy of Jonathan Merrill, HT Medical Ind., Rockville, MD).

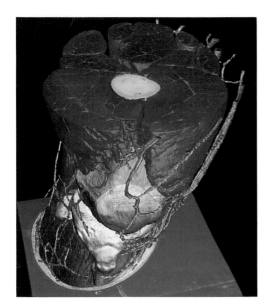

FIGURE 5.12. Near photo-realistic virtual knee (Courtesy of Dr. Victor Spitzer, University of Colorado Medical Center, Denver, CO).

FIGURE 5.13. Gunshot
wound of the thigh
(Courtesy of Dr. Scott Delp,
Musculographics,
Evanston, IL).

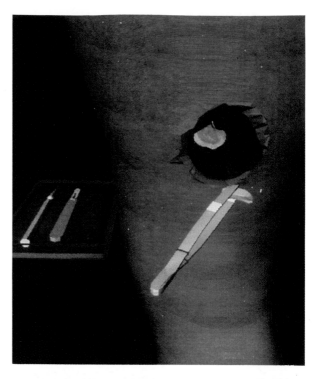

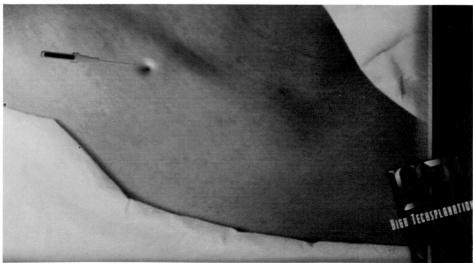

FIGURE 5.14. Central venous catheter simulator (Courtesy of Dr. Gerry Higgens,
HT Medical Ind., Rockville, MD).

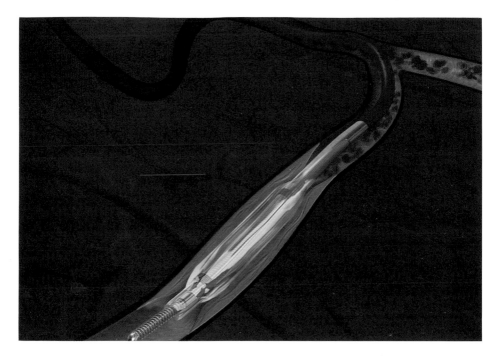

FIGURE 5.15. Virtual catheters used in endovascular simulators. (Courtesy of Mr. Kevin McGovern, CineMEd, Ind., Woodbury, CT).

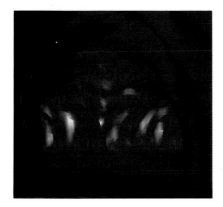

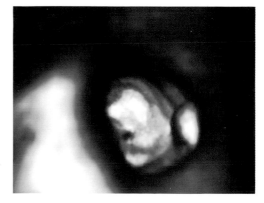

FIGURE 5.16. View of a virtual bronchoscopy (Courtesy of Dr. David Vining, Bowman Gray Medical Center, Winston-Salem, NC).

FIGURE 5.17. View of a virtual colonoscopy (Courtesy of Dr. Sandy Napel, Stanford Medical Center, Palo Alto, CA).

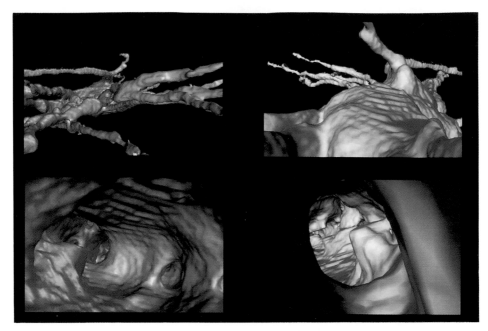

FIGURE 5.19. View of a virtual ganglion (Courtesy of Dr. Richard Robb, Mayo Clinic, Rochester, MN).

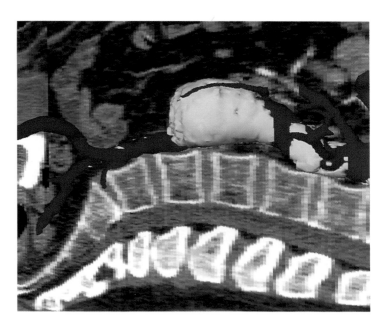

FIGURE 5.20.
Pre-operative
planning of aortic
reconstruction
(Courtesy of
Dr. Joseph Rosen,
Dartmouth
Medical Center,
Lebannon, NH).

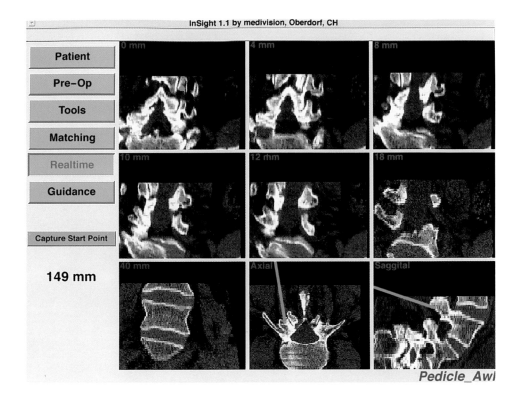

FIGURE 7.2. Realtime Trajectory.

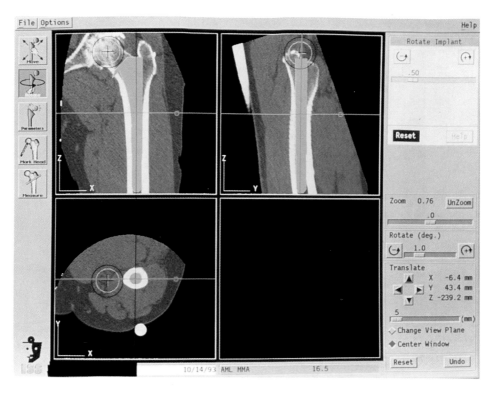

FIGURE 7.5. ORTHODOC™ preoperative planning.

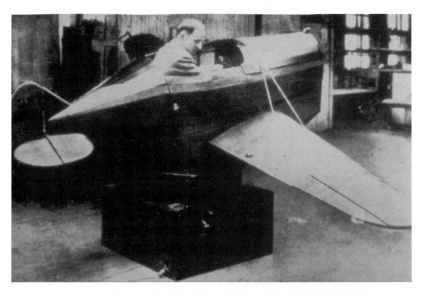

FIGURE 5.7. First flight simulator, located in Edwin Link's garage. (Courtesy of CAE-Link archives).

simulator was a carnival ride, training upon it was able to reduce crash landings in the dark or bad weather by over 90%. The point is that we do not have to wait for surgical simulators to become ultra-realistic, like the B-2 bomber simulator (Fig. 5.8) in order to obtain enormous training value. When questioned, B-2 pilots claim they prefer the simulator because it is more realistic that flying the actual aircraft—they are able to perform maneuvers they would not dare try on the actual aircraft, and thereby better learned exactly where the "edge of the envelop" is.

Out of these modest scientific accomplishments, virtual reality for surgical simulation and medical training began in the late 1980s when Drs. Scott Delp[5] and Joseph Rosen created one of the first virtual reality systems to investigate alternative surgical procedures (tendon transplants) of the lower leg (Fig. 5.9). In 1991 Satava and Lanier[6] created the first abdominal surgery simulator (Fig. 5.10),

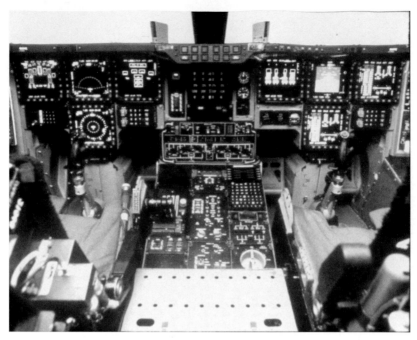

FIGURE 5.8. Cockpit of B-2 bomber flight simulator (courtesy of Dave Hood, Northrup Grumman, Pico Rivera, CA).

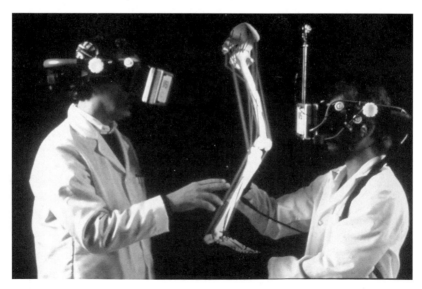

FIGURE 5.9. Virtual leg for preoperative planning of tendon transplantation (courtesy of Dr. Joseph Rosen, Dartmouth Medical Center, Lebannon, NH).

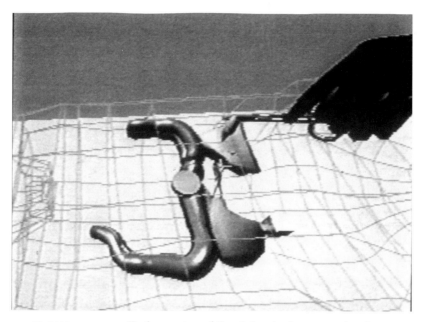

FIGURE 5.10. Early version of the abdominal surgery simulator.

using images of organs created in a simple graphics drawing program. These images were neither realistic nor highly interactive, but the simulator provided the opportunity to fly around and through the anatomy and to "practice" a surgical procedure with virtual instruments. Within 18 months, Jonathan Merrill[7] of High Techsplanations created a highly sophisticated graphic representation of the human torso (Fig. 5.11), with organs that had physical properties such as bending or stretching when pushed and pulled, or edges retracting when cut. The most significant landmark event was the 1994 release of National Library of Medicine's "Visible Human Project" under Dr. Michael Ackerman, which provided anatomic images that were reconstructed from an actual person's dataset. The virtual cadaver was created by Drs. Victor Spitzer and David Whitlock[8] of the University of Colorado from 1871 slices, 1 mm thick, which were accurately registered in three complete datasets: CT scan, MRI scan, and photographs from cryosections

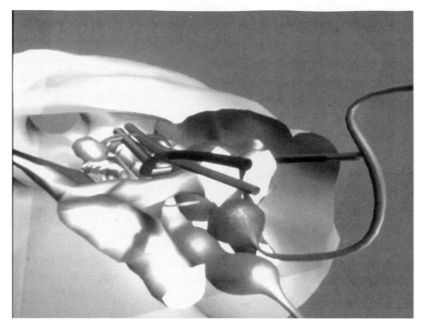

FIGURE 5.11. Second-generation surgical simulator, with tissue properties (courtesy of Jonathan Merrill, HT Medical Inc., Rockville, MD).

that had been digitized and stored in the computer. In rendering the images, there was near photorealism (Fig. 5.12); however, there were no properties because the entire power of the computer was used in portraying the image. Later that same year, Dr. Scott Delp used the Visible Human leg to create a Limb Trauma Simulator (Fig. 5.13). The image did not look as realistic as the Visible Human because so much computer power was used for the tissue properties, bleeding, wounding, and instrument interaction that a less realistic visual image resulted. Nevertheless, this model permitted debridement of the wound, removal of bone fragments, and stopping of hemorrhage. The purpose of this simulator is to decrease the number of animals that need to be wounded in order to train physicians and medics in the essentials of combat casualty care and trauma management; the system was installed as part of the curriculum in the combat casualty care training program of the Special Operations Command Medical Training Center, Ft. Bragg, NC, in

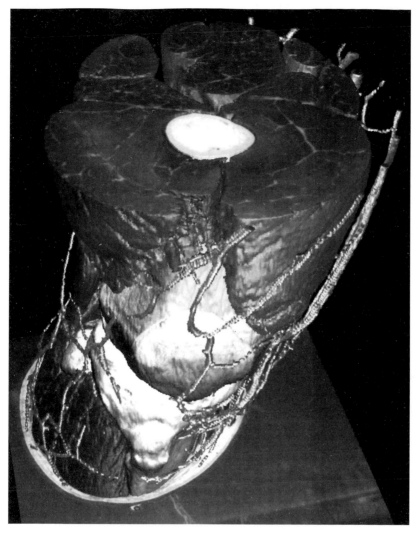

FIGURE 5.12. Near-photorealistic virtual knee (courtesy Dr. Victor Spitzer, University of Colorado Medical Center, Denver).

January 1997. In 1995 Dr. Jeffrey Levy constructed a surgical simulator for hysteroscopy. This system incorporated a haptic device for the hysteroscopic instruments and imported patient specific anatomy and pathology. Now for the first time, surgeons can practice on exactly the same virtual pathology that they would encounter in their patient. When the anatomy is not extremely

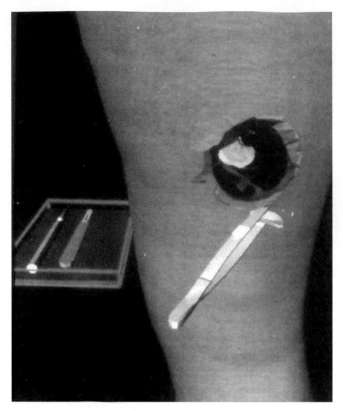

FIGURE 5.13. Gunshot wound of the thigh (courtesy of Dr. Scott Delp, Musculographics, Evanston, IL).

complex, a near-photorealistic image, with full tissue properties and haptic input can be achieved, such as the central venous catheter placement simulator by Gerry Higgins[9] of HT Medical Inc. (Fig. 5.14). And within the field of catheter-based endovascular therapy, simulators of catheter systems with balloon angioplasty and stent placement are being developed (Fig. 5.15).

As surgical simulators mature and develop, they must be continuously evaluated for effectiveness and value added. Johnston et al. have performed a surgical task analysis to determine the efficacy of training on simulators.[10] Employing the analytical tools of training transfer, used to evaluate pilot and astronaut training in virtual

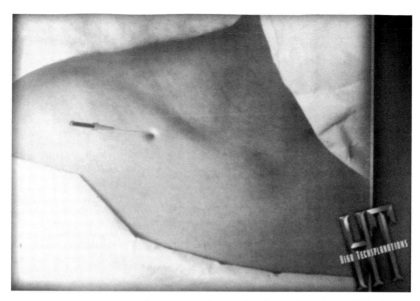

FIGURE 5.14. Central venous catheter simulator (courtesy of Dr. Gerry Higgins, HT Medical Inc., Rockville, MD).

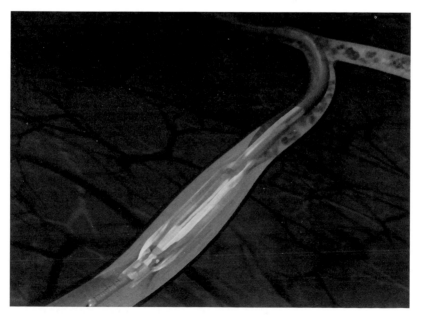

FIGURE 5.15. Virtual catheters used in endovascular simulators (courtesy of Kevin McGovern, CineMEd, Inc, Woodbury, CT).

environments, they obtained objective data to quantify the effectiveness and impact of simulators on surgical training.

In training transfer measurements, the time and accuracy of a task completed after one hour of simulation training is compared with the time and accuracy of the same task learned in a real situation. Initial results show substantial effectiveness: Training transfer of 28%–35% for surgical procedures learned on a simulator. Although these figures have proved to be higher for tasks learned with flight simulators—which produce training transfer of 48%–55%—one can expect the figures for surgical training simulators to rise to the same level when the surgical simulators become more sophisticated and realistic. When translated into hours of practice, these figures suggest that for every hour that a surgeon trains on a simulator, he will learn as much as 28%–35% of an hour (about 20 minutes) spent training on animals or patients.

An added benefit of virtual surgical training stems from a potential reduction in the number of animals sacrificed during medical education. While it is unlikely that animals and cadavers will ever be entirely eliminated from surgical and medical training, it may be possible to minimize their use.

Surgical simulators will soon prove their worth as educational tools, when the representational systems become more realistic, sufficient evidence documents simulator efficacy, and system costs fall enough to make them cost effective.

Along with the use of virtual environments for simulators is the emerging field of virtual endoscopy. Initial work was started simultaneously by Bill Lorensen of GE Medical, Ferenc Jolesz and Ron Kikinis of Brigham Women's Hospital,[11] Sandy Napel of Stanford University Medical Center, and David Vining of Bowman Gray Medical Center.[12] Virtual endoscopy refers to acquiring 3-D images from a patient with a CT, MRI, or ultrasound, and then "segmenting" the individual organs, neurovascular structures, and tissues from one another in order to "render" the patient in 3-D as a computer-generated "virtual patient." Thus what is seen on the video monitor is a 3-D representation of the patient's anatomy, which can be rotated, sliced, made transparent, cross-sectioned or viewed in any imaginable way. However, if sophisticated visualization algorithms (like those used by cruise missiles for flight planning and tracking) are applied, the virtual organs can be "flown through." The resultant image is exactly the same as if an endoscopic view were obtained by a video endoscope. Early works include virtual bronchoscopy (Fig. 5.16) and colonoscopy (Fig. 5.17). The next generation included "flights" through areas not possible with endoscopes, such as the inner ear (Fig. 5.18) and celiac ganglion (Fig. 5.19). Not only can the internal luminal views be obtained, but

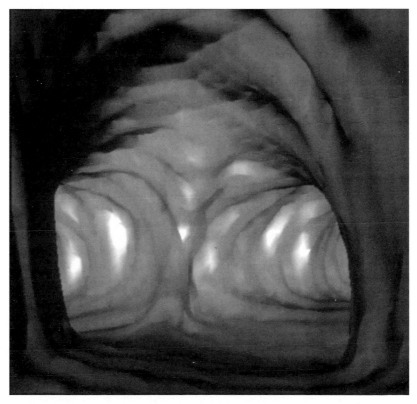

FIGURE 5.16. View of a virtual bronchoscopy (courtesy of Dr. David Vining, Bowman Gray Medical Center, Winston-Salem, NC).

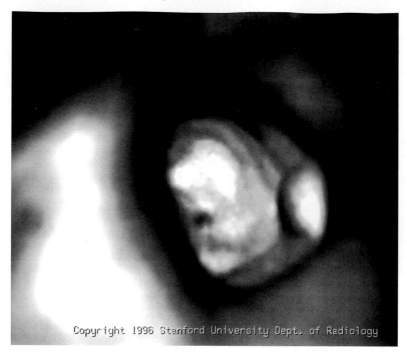

FIGURE 5.17. View of a virtual colonoscopy (courtesy of Dr. Sandy Napel, Stanford Medical Center, Palo Alto, CA).

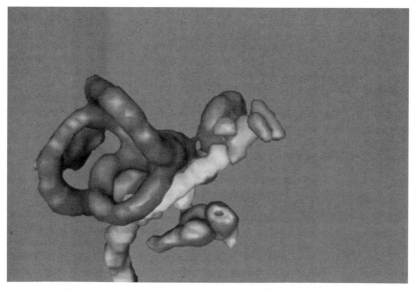

FIGURE 5.18. View of a virtual inner ear (courtesy of Drs. Ron Kinkinis and Ferenc Jolesz, Brigham Women's Hospital, Boston, MA).

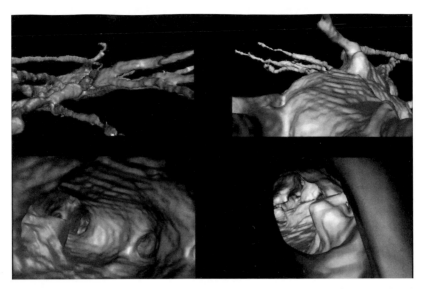

FIGURE 5.19. Views of a virtual ganglion (courtesy of Dr. Richard Robb, Mayo Clinic, Rochester, MN).

should a disease or cancer be encountered, the perspective can be flown "through the walls" to the outside of the structure in order to visualize penetration of the wall into the surrounding tissues or even nodal involvement. The technology now permits visualization of internal structures by noninvasive imaging techniques rather than the traditional minimally invasive endoscopic techniques at a level that is adequate only for anatomic distortions (cancers, polyps, ulcers, etc.) to a resolution of 1 mm accuracy, but not subtle changes of some disease states such as inflammation flat plaquelike lesions. With the use of other imaging modalities, such as infrared or PET, information about physiologic or functional disturbances may be acquired and fused with the anatomic display from CT or MRI to give information not otherwise available today. Using this technique of "data fusion," Mike Burrows of Engineering Anima-tion, Inc. is matching the textures of the photographic dataset to Houndsfield units of the CT scan and creating a "look-up table" that will permit the 3-D anatomy from a patient's CT scan to have not only anatomic accuracy but the correct texture to permit diagnosis. Vascular surgeons are using 3-D models of their patient's aortic aneurysm in order to do preoperative planning (Fig. 5.20). These initial efforts with image acquisition and reconstruction are the first steps in providing the total spectrum of patient care, as described in the previous chapters. In addition to diagnosis, this 3-D image can also be used for patient education and counseling, preoperative planning, virtual prototyping, surgical simulation to try different approaches to the surgical procedure, interoperative navigation, and postoperative follow-up.

Since the beginning of virtual environments as scientific tools, there has been the implementation of 3-D visualizations for prototyping instruments, equipment, and architectural spaces. There are a number of efforts to design the "operating environment of the future"[12] using virtual reality (Fig. 5.21). The advantages are obvious.

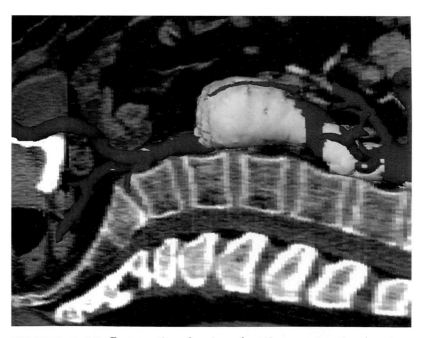

FIGURE 5.20. Preoperative planning of aortic reconstruction (courtesy of Dr. Joseph Rosen, Dartmouth Medical Center, Lebannon, NH).

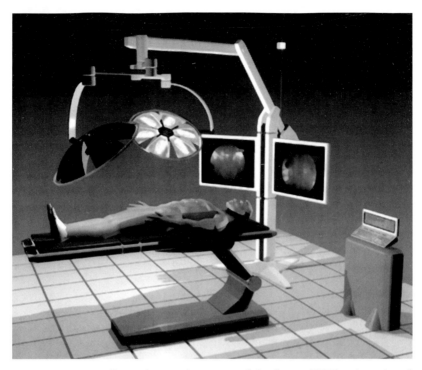

FIGURE 5.21. Operating environment of the future (OEF) using virtual reality (courtesy of Dave Hood, Northrup Grumman, Pico Rivera, CA).

Since it is unknown where minimally invasive therapy is taking us, the room can be designed to incorporate many modalities for surgery, imaging, catheter-based procedures, stereotactic navigation, and energy-directed therapies, to name a few. It would be impossible to build a room to incorporate all these modalities today without numerous trade-offs, revisions, and compromises. By first having the design in a virtual environment, all the various participants such as physicians, nurses, materiel managers, and safety inspectors can view, "walk around," and try out the room. The effect of adding a piece of equipment, or changing the wall, doors, or electrical outlets, can be evaluated over and over again until the room design is optimized. Then the room could be built, without previously gone through numerous iterations of building, tearing down, and rebuilding. There can be the exploration of new or developing technologies that are not available today but will soon be available, such as the large flat panel displays (also Fig. 5.21) or direct digital radiography, providing the chance to plan for future implementation even before the equipment is purchased. The important issues of human interface technology and ergonomics can be explored, especially considering the pervasiveness of communications and the ability to import information into the environment from anywhere in the world. Dr. Suzanne Weghorst of the University of Washington's Human Interface Technology Lab (HIT Lab) is exploring some of the difficult questions of human interface technology in a virtual emergency room. Should digital X rays be transmitted to the monitor on a wall, similar to current view boxes, or should they overlay the patient like "X-ray vision" or be suspended in an arbitrary position in the field of view? A virtual environment provides the opportunity to try out these and many other alternative possibilities.

While it is true that virtual reality and surgical simulators are here, it is also true that we are a long way from replacing the real world by the virtual. There are major advances required in order to bring the level of visual fidelity that approaches photorealism. Not only must the image be of very high resolution, but it must be rendered in real time (at least 30 frames a second). Physical and physiologic properties must be added to the anatomy. All of these require computers with much greater capability than exists today. Yet computers are continuing to have greater power so this is a temporary delay. There needs to be further research in the area of the sense of touch and haptic devices, so that tissues "feel" realistic. And most important, the core curriculum, training plans, and evaluation of the educational content must be in place when the technology is mature.

It should be obvious that virtual reality is many things. It is an imaginary computer-generated world where we can learn about the real world by interactive experimentation or practice difficult and complex problems through simulation. It is also the interface, the way we interact with information as if the bits and bytes were real objects. Since we are just on the threshold, there is a sense of elation at the challenge of the difficult barriers that must be overcome to realize the richness of high-fidelity virtual environments.

REFERENCES

1. Barfield W, Furness TA: Virtual Environments and Advanced Interface Design. New York: Oxford University Press, 1995:4–5.

2. Sutherland IE: "Computer displays." In *Sci. Am.* (1970) 222:57–81.

3. Fisher SS, McGreevy MM, Humphries J, Robinett W: "Virtual environment display system." In Crow F, Pizer S (ed.); *Proc of the Workshop on Interactive 3-D Graphics* (1986) 1:1–12.

4. Ellis SR: "Pictoral communication: Pictures and the synthetic environment." In Ellis SR (ed.), *Pictoral Communication in Virtual and Real Environments*, 2d ed. Washington: Taylor and Francis, 1993:22–40.

5. Delp SL, Zajac FR: "Force and moment generating capacity of lower limb muscles before and after tendon lengthening." *Clin Ortho Rel Res* (1992) 284:247–59.

6. Satava RM: "Virtual reality surgical simulator: The first steps." *Surg Endosc* (1993) 7:203–05.

7. Merril JR, Merril GL, Raju R, et al: "Photorealistic interactive 3-D graphics in surgical simulation." In Satava RM, Morgan K, et al. (eds.) *Interactive Technology and the New Medical Paradigm for Health Care.* Washington DC: IOS Press, 244–252.

8. Spitzer VM, Whitlock DG: "Electronic imaging of the human body: Data storage and interchange format standards." In Vannier MW, Yates RE, Whitestone JJ (eds.) *Proc Electronic Imaging of the Human Body Working Group* March 9–11, 1992:66–68.

9. Meglan DA, Raju R, Merril GL, Merril JR, Nguyen BH, Swamy SN, Higgins GA: "Teleos virtual environment for simulation-based surgical education." In Satava RM, Morgan K, et al. (eds.) *Interactive Technology and the New Medical Paradigm for Health Care.* Washington: IOS Press, 1995:346–51.

10. Johnston R, Bhoyrul S, Way L, Satava RM, et al: Assessing a virtual reality surgical skills simulator in Sieburg HF, Weghorst S, Morgan K, (eds.) *Health Care in the Information Age.* Washington: IOS Press, 1996:608–617.

11. Lorensen WE, Jolesz FA, Kikinis R: "The exploration of cross-sectional data with a virtual endoscope." In Satava RM, Morgan K, et al. (eds.) *Interactive Technology and the New Medical Paradigm for Health Care.* Washington: IOS Press, 1995:221–230.

12. Vining DN, Padhani AR, Wood S, et al.: "Virtual bronchoscopy: A new perspective for viewing the treacheobronchial tree." *Radiol* (1993) 189:438.

13. Kaplan K, Hunter I, Durlach NI, Schodek KL, Rattner D: "A virtual environment for a surgical room of the future." In Satava RM, Morgan K, et al. (eds.), *Interactive Technology and the New Medical Paradigm for Health Care.* Washington: IOS Press, 1995:161–67.

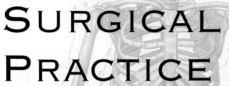

SURGICAL
PRACTICE

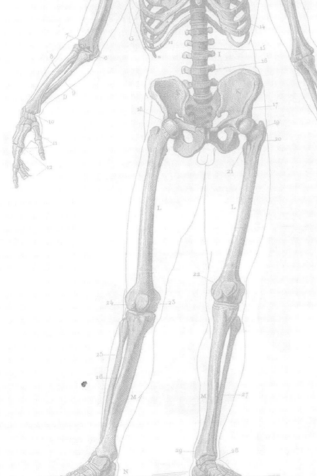

IMAGE-GUIDED PROCEDURES AND THE OPERATING ROOM OF THE FUTURE

FERENC A. JOLESZ, M.D.
AND RON KIKINIS, M.D.

I. INTRODUCTION

The ever-increasing need for enhanced visualization during interventional radiology and minimally invasive surgical procedures demands refinement of imaging modalities and image representation methods. The use of preoperative planning for selecting optimal surgical strategies and lifelike simulation of invasive procedures not only facilitates the training of surgeons and radiologists and encourages rehearsal of the procedures, but also substantiates the fundamental role of image guidance in the actual execution of the plan. Establishing this simulated procedural environment is a critical step for creating an image-based virtual reality. Intraoperative image guidance is based on the functional integration of this virtual three-dimensional information and the corresponding real anatomy of the patient within the same frame of reference. Links between these two corresponding components are realized by com-

Cybersurgery: Advanced Technologies for Surgical Practice,
Edited by Richard M. Satava, M.D.
ISBN 0-471-15874-7   Copyright © 1998 by Wiley-Liss, Inc.

bining image-to-patient registration and by tracking instruments within the operational field. These are the key ingredients of frameless stereotactic targeting methods, which capitalize on the interactive control of image planes and exploit the full information content of the virtual three-dimensional space.

Concurrent display of video images of the patient's exposed anatomy and the corresponding, preoperatively reconstructed three-dimensional information has already been demonstrated.[17] By merging the view of the exposed surgical field with the reconstructed surface representation of three-dimensional images, and in some cases with the correlated mapping of functional physiology of the cortex, has provided sufficient control of neurosurgical procedures even in high-risk areas. Parallel, comparative videoscopic images have been demonstrated with virtual endoscopic display of CT and magnetic resonance imaging (MRI) data in cross-sectional, surface, or volume presentation. The interactive matching of these views can improve both visualization and orientation during endoscopic interventions.

Because the use of preoperative images for intraoperative image guidance is limited by the potential changes in the anatomy during invasive procedures, real-time intraoperative imaging may become necessary. Advances in imaging technology and high-performance computing now allow us to combine and integrate near-real-time, volumetric images with frameless stereotactic, interactive localization methods while performing image-guided therapy.[13]

II. IMAGE-GUIDED THERAPY

The nondiagnostic use of cross-sectional imaging modalities is limited. The most frequently used interventional radiological procedure is percutaneous biopsy, which is essentially a diagnostic procedure. Image-guided therapy is a new, emerging field that has a close relationship to interventional radiology, minimally-invasive surgery, and computer-assisted visualization. Image guidance for minimally-invasive surgical and interventional therapeutic procedures is necessitated by the spatial restrictions of direct visual control.

While most of the surgical and interventional radiological procedures are executed within a well-defined operational volume, the anatomical details of this volume are not perceived by the operator. This is due to the fact that potential access routes are limited to minimize tissue damage. This limits the "navigational freedom" of the operator. Furthermore, the visualization of the anatomy is limited to the exposed surfaces, beyond which the human eye cannot penetrate. Imaging modalities can complement direct visualization of the surgeon or interventional radiologist by providing intraoperative image guidance. This can be achieved by image data obtained preoperatively and, after appropriate registration, displayed intraoperatively using computer visualization techniques. Alternatively, procedures can be monitored and controlled by intraoperative, real-time imaging when direct visualization can be updated and complemented by simultaneously-acquired image data from the same spatial location. In both cases, interactive control of the image planes, with or without tracking the instruments, is necessary. Intraoperative control of therapeutic procedures (thermal ablations, interstitial drug- or chemotherapy, etc.) requires imaging methods with specific sensitivity to the physical changes induced by the particular interventions.

Intraoperative image-guidance has the following components:

LOCALIZATION AND TARGETING

The primary role of imaging in surgical or other therapeutic procedures is the definition of target volume and its localization in relationship to surrounding anatomic structures. This spatial information can be used to plan access routes and trajectories and to approach the target with appropriate instruments or devices.

1. *Target Definition.* There is sparse and inconclusive data on the role of diagnostic imaging modalities in defining tumor margins. Comparison of imaging techniques and spatially-registered histology is necessary to estimate the capabilities of imaging in defining tumor boundaries and providing guidance for surgical excisions or ablations. If intraoperative image guidance can provide exact definition of tumor margins, the efficiency of surgical procedures can be improved significantly.

2. *Trajectory Selection.* Research in the area of surgical planning and simulation is essential for the development of image-guided surgery. Trajectory planning is the principal element of this process. Biopsy is the basic procedure, since most of the more complex surgeries or interventions can be described as multiple trajectories.

3. *Registration.* For intraoperative guidance, cross-sectional and 3-D reconstructed images have to be presented and displayed in a close approximation to the directly visualized anatomy. There is significant room for improving current registration methods by using more complex automated technologies. Especially important is the use of various optical methods, including video-based and laser-scanning techniques.

4. *Instrument and Tip Tracking.* Positional information of needles, catheters, and surgical instruments is important for registration, localization, and targeting and to interactively obtain or recall images. There are various sensors (optical, electromagnetic, ultrasonic, etc.) that can be attached to instruments and provide continuous spatial localization during interventional and surgical procedures. There is an alternative way to follow the movement of devices within the operational volume using real-time imaging and image processing.

5. *Stereotaxy.* Both frame-based and frameless stereotaxy should be introduced by image-guided therapy as a basic and necessary concept. Minimally-invasive approaches require more accurate sampling of tumors that can be treated *in situ.* Not only biopsies, but also other trajectories, should be defined by interactive image acquisition and by identifying appropriate reference frame(s) in order to transfer image data from one frame to the other.

MONITORING

There is a need to define the temporal resolution requirements for image-guided therapy procedures. Depending on the task, the requirements are variable and more-or-less adaptable. The physical characteristics of the specific imaging modalities and the dynamic properties of the monitored procedures should be considered. For those interventions in which the changes are developing within a volume (i.e., thermal ablations and interstitial drug injection) single-slice monitoring is not appropriate. Therefore, in most cases, temporal resolution should be defined for multislice volumetric monitoring. One of the most important research needs is related to the display of dynamic image data, especially if the changes are in 3-D. Real-time image processing and high-performance computing are necessary to monitor changes occurring within image volumes.

CONTROL

Control of destructive energy deposition is essential to develop effective and safe treatment protocols. Interstitial laser therapy, cryoablation, and high-intensity focused ultrasound treatment all require imaging and can be potentially controlled by image-derived data. The temperature sensitivity of imaging techniques should be combined with tissue characterization of the thermal damage to achieve full control of these procedures.

INTEGRATION OF IMAGING WITH THERAPY

One of the most challenging tasks is the integration of imaging methods with therapeutic procedures. This integration includes feedback systems among output devices and image information, computer-assisted, image-controlled surgical tools, robotic arms, and instruments. Compatibility of various interventional and surgical tools and imaging systems is important, especially in the case of MR-guided therapy.

III. INFRASTRUCTURE REQUIREMENTS FOR IMAGE-GUIDED THERAPY

A program that focuses on multiple aspects of image guidance requires a complex infrastructure. A systematic approach should address the main ingredients of image guidance: visualization, localization, access, and control.[11]

SURGICAL PLANNING

In traditional surgical planning, which is a direct continuation of the diagnostic work-up, it has been the role of the radiologist to provide the most complete anatomical description of the region or tissue volume under investigation and to facilitate the use of these images to support the procedure. For diagnostic purposes, cross-sectional images are usually sufficient. When 3-D visualization represents a useful addition for diagnosis, as in complex spine or pelvic fractures, time is not a limiting factor. Similarly, 3-D image reconstruction for surgical planning and simulation occurs during the preoperative phase. This makes the length of time required for reconstruction of the cross-sectional images is more or less irrelevant. However, if 3-D images are to be obtained intraoperatively, real-time or close-to-real-time image processing is required. The goal of modern surgical planning is to use computerized image-processing tools for both preoperative planning and near-real-time intraoperative image visualization.

There are several components of this process that are going on in parallel, in order to develop new processing algorithms, integrate new algorithms into the existing software environment, and to apply these image-processing tools to address clinical questions. Interdisciplinary teams consisting of radiologists, computer scientists, clinicians, and basic researchers are developing customized protocols and processing pipelines to answer medical questions in a quantitative way. In addition, there are unique visualization requirements in different surgical specialties such as craniofacial surgery, neurosurgery, orthopedic surgery, abdominal surgery, and endoscopic surgery. The overall goal is to develop a rich and robust software environment capable of handling a variety of image modalities and clinical questions.

Computer algorithms are developed for applications that initially had no real-time requirements. High-end workstations and supercomputers provide increasingly more speed, as well as the flexibility to explore multiple algorithmic approaches in parallel. Due to the rapidly increasing performance available on desktop systems, we expect that the work performed now on the supercomputer systems will become possible on desktop systems within a few years.

IMAGE-PROCESSING TOOLS

The creation of the 3-D models first involves the so-called *segmentation* of the images, or the computational process initiated with the identification or selection of different tissue classes.[3,20] If automated, segmentation requires high-performance computers and high-speed computation to allow almost immediate display of the color-coded digital anatomy. This is followed by 3-D rendering of the data using various display techniques. After these initial steps, the 3-D images have to be projected onto the corresponding anatomy of the patient to be used for localization. This process, called *registration*, is extremely important for many image-guided procedures. Without accurate image-to-patient registration, images cannot provide an exact roadmap for interventional or surgical procedures. The development of MRI techniques has increased the potential to accomplish these basic steps and apply them in a near-real-time environment.

INTERACTIVE IMAGE MANIPULATION

Sensors attached to instruments have created new capabilities in tools. Surgical or interventional tools like needles, forceps, and scalpels can be tracked within the image space, and their position can be used as the reference for acquiring various image planes, choosing view angles, or performing other interactive image manipulations.[1] This concept of interactive image acquisition is a change for diagnostic radiologists who are accustomed to fixed image planes and projections and do not usually need to relate the reference frame from one image set to another. However, stereotactic procedures, with and without the use of frames, require establishment of reference frames, assessment of the correspondence between them, and knowledge of a tool's position in relationship to the surrounding anatomy.

Real-time imaging can be combined with frameless stereotaxy. In the open magnet system a "frameless stereotactic" method for localization and targeting[13] can be performed. The basic concept is that the tools (in the case of biopsy, the needle holder) can be localized by attaching two flashing, light-emitting diodes (LEDs) to their surface. These LEDs produce invisible infrared beams that are detected by their sensors and localized by simple triangulation. The computer essentially has continuous positional information about the tip and about the alignment of the needle holder's axis within the space.

This optical localizing device is an integral part of the MR system (Fig. 6.1). It allows tracking of any tool or instrument within the system if the direct optical link between the LEDs and the sensors, located above the imaging field, can be established. Images can be either generated according to the position of an instrument

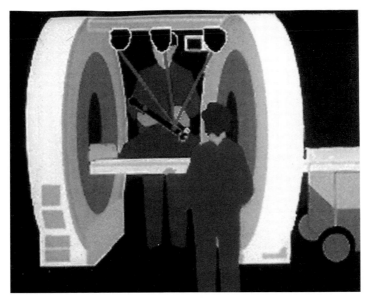

FIGURE 6.1. Interactive image guidance within the intraoperative MRI system: There are infrared light-emitting diodes (LEDs) attached to the instruments. The positions of these LEDs are tracked with three infrared-sensitive cameras. The location and axis of the acquired scan planes is determined by the location of the LEDs within the magnet.

in conventional axial-coronal-sagittal planes or used like an ultrasound (US) transducer with the images generated along the axis of the optically tracked tool. Image planes defined by this axis can be changed, however, without moving the tool itself. Using audio communications with the technologist, the physician can request images in the 0, 90 plane (referenced to the room) or in the plane perpendicular to the axis of the tool. Positioning the optically tracked tools and selecting the related image planes provides an interactive way to localize targets, define trajectories, and review alternative access routes. If the defined plane goes through both the entry and target point and a review of the anatomy shows no problems, the needle can be advanced to the target. This one-step localization and targeting using image guidance is the essential feature of frameless stereotaxy.

In the open magnet there is no need for a multi-step process to register images with patient anatomy, to define trajectories, and perform a biopsy. Instead, the radiologist interactively scans through the image volume until the appropriate image/trajectory is found. Then the needle, which is also under continuous image visibility, can be advanced. Since the needle holder is localized during biopsy, the images will be in the same plane as the needle (although some distortion due to bending of the biopsy needle is possible).

VIDEO REGISTRATION FOR INTRAOPERATIVE GUIDANCE

One form of possible intraoperative image guidance uses previously acquired image data that is registered to the individual patient's anatomy. The surface of the computerized image of the patient is aligned with a visual image of the same person acquired with a simple video camera.[17] The alignment is based on matching of various anatomic features: nose aligned with nose, lip with lip, and ears and eyes with ears and eyes. This process is done with a video-mixer which overlays the computer-generated 3-D graphics with the video image of the patient from the surgeon's vantage point. After the face is registered, the internal structures, like the brain surface, can be superimposed upon the skull. This *video registration* allows definition of the cortical anatomy of the brain to be superimposed on the skull surface.[13,17] Using video registration, we can see the image of the tumor overlaid on the patient in any stage of the neurosurgical process (Fig. 6.2). This approach has served in dozens of neurosurgical and craniofacial procedures. Its main limitation is that we are using a camera with a fixed position. If the surgeon is not closely aligned with the camera's viewpoint, we run into problems with parallaxis. This effect is most severe with deep lying tumors. The method is well suited for the planning of craniotomies and in the case of tumors close to the surface. More recently cortical veins were used to realign the image data after per-

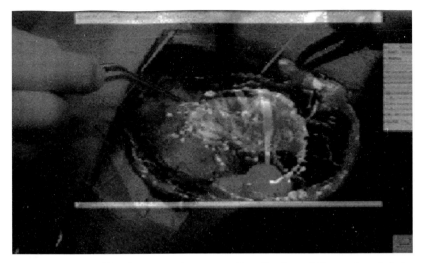

FIGURE 6.2. Simultaneous intraoperative display of the real and "virtual" view of the surgical field. On the same monitor are overlayed the video image and the surface rendering of MRI data. Registration of the computer-generated data to the patient's anatomy is achieved by the preoperative matching of the patient skin surface with the skin surface reconstructed from images. Further improvement in registration is possible intraoperatively by matching the visible cortical blood vessels with their "virtual" counterparts obtained from MR angiogram.

forming the craniotomy.[18] The utilization of local anatomy (in relation to the tumor) for registration purposes can result in very good overlays.

In order to replace the qualitative registration ("by eyeballing") with a more quantitative approach, a new automated registration method has been introduced that utilizes laser surface scanning instead of the camera images.[7] This will allow the computer to perform the registration in a quantitative way. This method allows fast frameless stereotaxy without touching the patient. In order to deal with the parallaxis problem, interfacing with the OR microscope equipped with stereo cameras and a computer-controlled overlay system is necessary. This device will put the camera systems into the same line of view as the surgeon's.

A significant problem with this intraoperative guidance approach is that it uses images acquired prior to the surgery and thus cannot show any potential changes that may occur during the surgery. In the case of brain surgery, the removal of some cerebrospinal fluid, repositioning of the head, brain swelling, or hemorrhage can all shift the brain structures from their original positions. Even greater shifts of anatomical structures can be expected during abdominal surgery. Here, updated image guidance correction is not possible, and error is more or less unavoidable. The promise of intraoperative imaging within an open magnet system is the continuous refreshment of the original image, so correction or reregistration will always be possible.

IV. MAGNETIC RESONANCE IMAGE–GUIDED THERAPY

Although various imaging modalities can provide some image guidance, MRI has the most potential for monitoring interventional and surgical procedures. Nearly all features of conventional MRI are already consistent with the requirements for ideal image guidance. MRI provides the best tissue characterization of any existing imaging modalities, and the resulting images are multiplanar and volumetric. In addition, MRI parameters have specific properties that can be useful in detecting temperature changes and tissue coagulation, which can be exploited in monitoring thermal ablations. MRI's flow sensitivity is applicable for vascular interventions. By using fast and ultrafast imaging or MR fluoroscopy with an interactive image display, MRI has the potential to be a real-time monitoring device.

Because of its high contrast and spatial resolution as well as multiplanar and functional capabilities, MRI has the most appeal for intraoperative monitoring and control of therapy. Open configuration magnets, which permit full access to the patient and are equipped with instrument-tracking systems, provide an interactive environment in which biopsies, endoscopic procedures, and minimally invasive interventions or surgeries are performed.[18] In addition, various thermal ablations with image-based control of energy deposition can be performed to exploit the intrinsic sensitivity of MRI to both temperature and tissue integrity.[14] Among these procedures, the noninvasive, MRI-guided focused ultrasound ablation has the most promising future and may replace some conventional surgeries.[4]

MRI has potential appeal to most of the minimally-invasive, minimal-access approaches. The most obvious role of MRI is in monitoring and controlling a variety of interstitial ablative methods, including thermal therapy (interstitial laser therapy, cryosurgery, focused ultrasound surgery). One of the fundamental requirements of MRI monitoring is the implementation of pulse sequences with spatial and temporal resolution as well as overall image quality suitable for the dynamic imaging tasks. In addition, magnet configurations need to allow greater access for the various interventional procedures to be executed. MR compatibility of instruments and devices should be addressed and therapeutic modalities need to be integrated with the MR system.

The spatial resolution of MRI, which can be extended into the submillimeter range, is appropriate for localizing and guiding therapy. MRI can acquire multiplanar and 3-D volume images directly, allowing full appreciation of important anatomical relationships. The temporal resolution of various fast and ultrafast imaging sequences permits a near-real-time viewing of physiological motions and the changes induced by interventional procedures.

A distinct advantage of MRI over the other imaging techniques is its ability to characterize functional and/or physical parameters of the treated tissue such as diffusion, perfusion, flow, and temperature. Using this information to depict tissue damage induced by various destructive energy sources, MRI has the unparalleled potential to monitor and control interventional or minimally invasive surgical procedures. The goal is to integrate therapeutic tools and

techniques into the armamentarium of MRI. From surgical planning through specialized imaging systems with minimally invasive
surgical applications, new methods are being developed and implemented. This new field of image-guided therapy will require extensive clinical development and evaluation.

The most important requirement for image guidance is the integration of the imaging system with various components of the therapeutic or surgical procedures. In conventional, closed-configura-
tion MRI systems there is no direct access to the patient, so
image-guided procedures cannot be done under MRI guidance. Ver-
tically open configuration magnets provide, in our opinion, the best
opportunities for MR-guided interventions because they allow full
access to the exposed anatomy of the patient. The physician can perform various procedures while standing or sitting between the two
components of the magnet system (Fig. 6.3).

A prototype of this MR imaging system[18] has been developed
by GE Medical Systems in collaboration with the MRI Division of
the Brigham and Women's Hospital in Boston where it is the center-
piece of the Interventional MRI Center. This center is the result of a
cross-fertilization between an operating room, interventional radiology suite, and a conventional MRI center. The image quality of
the MR Special Procedure System is comparable to that obtained on
the 0.5T clinical system. Images taken with the flexible transmit-re-
ceive (T–R) coils are of diagnostic quality and give sufficient detail
for most procedures. For larger anatomical regions, like the abdomen, the flexible coils cannot provide uniform signal intensity,
and without the body coil an entire cross section of the abdomen
cannot be obtained. In addition the homogeneous magnetic field
represents only a 30-cm diameter volume at the center of the magnet. Since the primary application of the system is interventional
not diagnostic, these characteristics do not create substantial problems. The MR interventional procedures usually follow a diagnostic
work-up; therefore, imaging is limited to the target volume during
the course of the biopsy or other intervention.

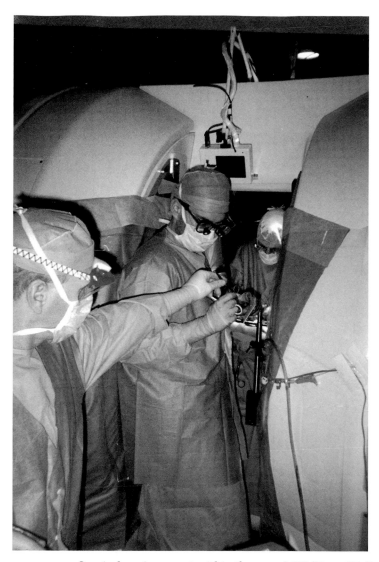

FIGURE 6.3. Surgical environment within the open MRI (Signa SP, General Electric Medical Systems). The integration of imaging and surgical tools has been accomplished, which allows the performance of various interventional and surgical procedures.

MRI-GUIDED BIOPSY

Traditionally stereotactic methods have been used only by neuro-
surgeons, but now the trend is to use the same principles for accurately localizing biopsy specimens throughout the entire body. Minimally-invasive therapies that remove or ablate tumors *in situ*
minimize the available material for pathology and destroy the original anatomic landmarks, especially tumor margins. The only solu-
tion is to define the biology of the tumor and localize its exact extent
in a series of precise biopsies under image guidance. This is the
main reason why the stereotactic approach to tumor diagnosis and
treatment is so important. The use of imaging systems, especially
MRI, resolves the conflict between the need for correct pathology
samples and minimally-invasive approaches. Using image fusion
techniques, like the combination of MRI with CT, PET, SPECT, or
angiography, can be extremely helpful in fully defining and anatomically characterizing the tumors.

There are relatively simple computer techniques primarily used
for surgical planning and simulation. Planning biopsy trajectories is
another critical part of image-guided intervention. In most cases the
biopsy trajectory is a straight line between the entry and the target
point. More complex surgical procedures can be described by multiple trajectories. Trajectory planning for all procedures is related to
optimizing access and reducing the damage to adjacent normal tissues. The knowledge of the corresponding anatomy is a basic requirement in all preplanned or real-time image-guided procedures.
In the near future real-time image processing and display will allow us to use computerized tools to improve visualization of the
anatomy during the interventional or surgical procedures.

MR-guided biopsies have been performed in open magnet systems with the combination of frameless stereotaxy with real-time
MRI.[19] The localization of tumors is achieved with interactive image
plane acquisition and targeting by using a needle icon. Near-real-
time (1–2 s) images demonstrate the needle advancement. The
planned or anticipated trajectory of the needle can be used for tar-

geting and later for comparing the path of the real needle with the planned trajectory. Review of the orthogonal planes related to the axis of the needle allows an appreciation of anatomy around the needle path. The near-real-time imaging offers an opportunity for correction and also replaces the depth measurement necessary for non-monitored cross-sectional biopsies.

A similar system has been utilized for brain biopsies.[16] Rather than the free-hand procedures used in the abdominal biopsies, a flexible arm was used with an attached needle holder to target the brain tumors and to maintain the trajectory angles during the needle placement. This procedure is distinguished from other frameless stereotactic methods as it utilizes real-time images for targeting.

VI. MRI-Guided Endoscopy

The combination of real-time MRI with various endoscopic techniques may provide the most important techniques for minimally invasive therapy. The access to internal structures via existing orifices and openings is relatively simple with various rigid or flexible endoscopes. Nevertheless, visualization through these devices is restricted to the internal surfaces of the organs. By complementing the videoscopic surface images with volumetric MRI, the endoscopist can appreciate the entire anatomy of the organ.

Several sinus endoscopic procedures were performed in open MRI system.[8] In this procedure the tracking device is attached to a pointer that can be used to point to structures within the visual field of the sinus endoscope. Images can then be made to demonstrate the location of the pointer tip relative to the surrounding anatomy. In the case of the paranasal sinuses, intraoperative imaging can adequately depict all "hidden" tissues that cannot be revealed by the endoscope.

MRI has also allowed a kind of virtual endoscopy to be developed.[9,14] Cross-sectional presentation precludes contiguous viewing of the inner wall, especially of tubular organs such as the bowel or blood vessels. To improve interpretation and exploration, surface-rendered images are derived from computer reconstructions to allow an endoscopy-like view of the inner surfaces. Various display methods and exploration strategies have been used to demonstrate simultaneous presentation of inner surfaces with anatomical structures that surround the visualized wall. Endoluminal images of intracerebral ventricles, paranasal sinuses, tracheobronchial tree, gastrointestinal tract, bladder and kidneys, and vessels have been displayed stereoscopically as virtual reality. During active exploration the operator has full control of navigation within the hollow organ, and "fly-through" within tubular organs is possible. By the tip-tracking approach mentioned below, we will be able to use these virtual endoscopy techniques for improved display even with flexible endoscopes.

VII. MRI-CONTROLLED THERMAL ABLATIONS

Further improvements in surgical strategies are related to optimizing access routes and controlling the spatial extent of destructive energies. Control of destructive energy deposition has been, until now, an unresolved problem in tumor treatment. This is especially true in the case of thermal ablative procedures. A direct measurement or mapping of tissue temperature distribution can only be done with multiple temperature-sensitive probes introduced into the tissue invasively. The number of thermocouples or temperature-sensitive fiber-optic devices is usually insufficient to monitor the spatiotemporal heat distribution. Furthermore, no imaging technique signals the end point of these thermal procedures (the phase transitions), which are consistent with lethal and irreversible tissue damage. Adequate monitoring of tissue temperature and temperature-induced tissue changes is necessary for controlling energy deposition. Repeated temperature-sensitive MRI sequences may fulfill this requirement.[9,14]

The role of MRI is twofold in imaging thermal surgery: to restrict the energy deposition to the target tissue by demonstrating the transient temperature elevation in the surrounding normal tissue, and to signal the irreversible phase transition within the target volume. Both the reversible changes within the normal tissue and irreversible phase transitions within the tumor tissue provide important information that can be used to control (terminate or continue) energy deposition. In this way MRI provides feedback for monitoring thermal ablations. Both experimental and clinical interstitial laser therapy, a typical high-temperature ablative procedure, has been controlled by continuous MR monitoring of the thermal-induced changes during energy delivery. MRI-guided laser treatment of brain and liver tumors has also been tested.[5,12,21]

Other kinds of thermal ablations can be controlled with MRI as well. Cryotherapy is a cold thermal method that uses a biopsy-like targeting and the introduction of a freezing probe into the tumor. The frozen tissue is clearly visible on MR images because of the change of tissue matter to solid ice crystal. Solid ice crystals give no measurable MR signal, and the expanding freezing zone on MRI is therefore represented by increasing signal void.[6,15]

The potentially most significant of the thermal ablative methods is focused ultrasound (FUS) heating. As opposed to the other two methods, FUS heating does not involve an invasive probe. The FUS beam is targeted by positioning a transducer outside the body and causing a tissue-killing energy dose to develop in a "hotpoint" within the body without causing any damage to surrounding or intervening tissue. There is no need for skin incision and spatial control is achieved by the motion of the transducer. MRI-guided FUS is the tumor ablation method of the twenty-first century. Because this procedure can be performed within the MRI system and the heat deposition can be both monitored and controlled by MRI, it has the most significant potential for tumor treatment.[2,4] Using relatively low energies, a slight but MRI detectable temperature elevation is induced at the focal point. The heat deposition causes no irreversible tissue damage, and therefore we are able to move the focal point on the desired target location without making any permanent changes. This process allows temperature-sensitive sequences to create MR images localizing the focal area. When targeting is completed, the energy level is increased, and the resulting higher temperature (60–90°C) causes the denaturing of the proteins. This type of energy delivery is safe and accurate within a few millimeters. It is possible to induce lesions as small as 1 mm using FUS. The spatial resolution of MRI systems therefore is comparable to the accuracy of the FUS system, which is as accurate as the hand of any good surgeon.

VIII. THE ROLE OF INTEGRATION IN IMAGE-GUIDED THERAPY

MRI-guided FUS is a good example of therapeutic devices being integrated with imaging systems. This integration is a prerequisite of image-guided therapy. Both localization and feedback control of the energy disposition call for a fully integrated system. We are entering a new area of medical applications of high technology. There are still unresolved problems, and the clinical efficacy of the techniques must be further tested. Nevertheless, the few cases already performed contribute to a feasibility study.

Image-guided therapy is an interdisciplinary field. Image guidance itself is a very general concept applicable to controlling many interventional procedures which will revolutionize the field of therapy. Various devices, including surgical robots, computer-assisted interventional tools, and energy delivery devices need image-derived information for feedback control of their actions. Not only radiologists, but surgeons, computer scientists, engineers, and physicists are contributing to the development of this exciting new field. There is also a need for strong collaboration between academic sites and the industry. Our ultimate goal is to take these superb technologies—the MRI, the therapy systems, and the computers—into the operating room of the next century.[11]

The vision of the operating room of the future is based on the fundamental concept of merging these exciting new technologies into an environment in which both surgery and interventional radiology can be performed with image guidance. The central role of imaging necessitates the principal involvement of a radiologist (both as imager and interventionalist) in this procedural environment. The next generation of medical imaging applications for surgical and interventional procedure planning and guidance has been developed. Successful integration of basic research and clinical work has already resulted in a number of cutting-edge technologies with direct clinical applications. The large, concentrated interdisciplinary effort, which brings together clinicians, surgeons, radiologists, computer scientists, and physicists will eventually change the way we approach patient care and health care in general.

REFERENCES

1. Bucholz RD, Smith KR, Henderson J, et al.: "Intraoperative localization using a three dimensional optical digitizer." *SPIE* (1993) 1894:312–322.
2. Cline HE, Hynynen K, Watkins RD, et al.: "A focused ultrasound system for MRI guided ablation." *Radiol* (1995) 195:176–180.
3. Cline HE, Lorensen WE, Kikinis R, Jolesz F: "Three-dimensional segmentation of MR images of the head using probability and connectivity." *JCAT* (1990) 14(6):1037–1045.
4. Cline HE, Schenck JF, Hynynen K, et al.: "MR-guided focused ultrasound surgery." *JCAT* (1992) 16:956–965.
5. Darkazani A, Hynynen K, Unger EC, Schenck JF: "On-line monitoring of ultrasonic surgery with MR imaging." *J Magn Reson Imag* (1993) 3:509–514.
6. Gilbert JC, Rubinsky B, Roos MS, et al.: "MRI-monitored cryosurgery in rabbit brain." *Magn Reson Imag* (1993) 11:1158–1164.
7. Grimson E, Lozano-Perez T, Wells W, et al.: "Automated registration for enhanced reality visualization in surgery." Proc First International Symposium on Medical Robotics and Computer Aided Surgery. Pittsburgh, 1994.
8. Hsu L, Jolesz FA, Fried MP. "Interactive MR-guided sinus endoscopy." *Radiol* (1995) 197(P):237.

9. Jolesz FA, Bleier AR, Jakab P, et al.: "MR imaging of laser tissue interaction." *Radiol* (1988) 168:249–253.

10. Jolesz FA, Lorensen WE, Kikinis R, et al.: "Virtual endoscopy: Three-dimensional rendering of cross-sectional images for endoluminal visualization." *Radiol* (1994) 193(P):469.

11. Jolesz FA, Shtern F: "The operating room of the future." *Invest Radiol* (1992) 27:236–238.

12. Khanm T, Bettag M, Ulrich F, et al.: "MR-imaging guided laser-induced interstitial thermotherapy in cerebral neoplasm." *JCAT* (1994) 18:519–532.

13. Kikinis R, Gleason LP, Lorensen W, et al.: Proc Third Conference on Visualization in Biomedial Computing. Rochester, MN: *SPIE*, 1994.

14. Matsumoto R, Mulkern RV, Hushek SG, Jolesz FA: "Tissue temperature monitoring for thermal intervention: A comparison of T1-weighted MR pulse sequences." *J Magn Reson Imag* (1993) 4:65–70.

15. Matsumoto R, Oshio K, Jolesz FA: "Monitoring of laser and freezing-induced ablation in the liver with T1 weighted MR imaging." *J Magn Reson Imag* (1996) 3:770–776.

16. Moriarty TM, Kikinis R, Jolesz FA, Black PMcL, Alexander E: "Magnetic resonance imaging therapy." *Neuro Clin North Am* (1996) 7(2):323–331.

17. Nakajima S, Atsumi H, Moriarty TM, Kikinis R, Jolesz FA, Black PMcL: "The use of cortical surface vessel registration for image-guided neurosurgery." Submitted to Neurosurg, May 1996.

18. Schenck JF, Jolesz Fa, Roemer PB, et al.: "Superconducting open-configuration MR imaging system for image-guided therapy." *Radiol* (1995) 195:805–814.

19. Silverman SG, Collick BD, Figueira MR, et al.: "Interactive biopsy in an open configuration interventional MRI system." *Radiol* (1995) 197:173–181.

20. Shenton ME, Kikinis R, Jolesz FA, et al.: "Left-lateralized temporal lobe abnormalities in schizophrenia and their relationship to thought disorder: A computerized quantitative MRI study." *NEJM* (1992) 326:604–612.

21. Vogl TJ, Muller PK, Hammerstingl, et al.: "Malignant liver tumors treated with MR imaging-guided laser-induced thermotherapy: Technique and prospective results." *Radiol* (1995) 196:257–265.

Computer-Aided Surgery

Anthony M. DiGioia, M.D.,
Bruce D. Colgan, M.S., and
Nancy Koerbel

I. Introduction

Recent advances in the fields of medical imaging, computer vision, and robotics have allowed computer-aided surgery to become a viable means of identifying and addressing clinical needs. Although these technologies have been applied in industry for over 20 years, the field of computer-aided surgery is still in its infancy. The medical community is only now beginning to see the benefit of extending such technology to the area of patient treatment through the collaboration and combined expertise of engineers, roboticists, surgeons, and computer scientists.

Applications for computer assistants, image-guided techniques, and robotics span a wide range of specialties from neurosurgery to orthopedics. The use of computer assistants and medical robots provides increased precision, dexterity, endurance, information, and insight that cannot be attained through use of traditional tools. These high-tech tools augment a surgeon's skill and judgment with such

Cybersurgery: Advanced Technologies for Surgical Practice,
Edited by Richard M. Satava, M.D.
ISBN 0-471-15874-7   Copyright © 1998 by Wiley-Liss, Inc.

beneficial qualities as greater accuracy and precision, and provide motion stability inherent only to a machine. The systems discussed here range from simulators and trainers, which never enter the operating suite, to fully autonomous robots, which perform actions independent of the surgeon. Most computer-aided surgery is still in the research and development phase, although some systems are FDA approved and currently in use. In addition several clinical trials are currently under way and scores of other systems are just entering the development phase.

II. BACKGROUND

Much of the early work of computer-assisted surgery centered on tumor stereotaxis (the location of bodily structures using coordinate systems) introduced by Clarke and Horseley nearly a century ago. The field has expanded to include specialties such as general surgery, neurosurgery, orthopedics, and otolaryngology. Recent technological developments have created 3-D imaging and real-time image-guided applications that were previously impossible, thus providing information to the surgeon both before and during surgery that was formerly unavailable. Projects such as CAMI (Computer-Assisted Medical Interventions) at Grenoble Hospital in France, MRCAS (Medical Robotics and Computer-Assisted Surgery) at Shadyside Hospital and Carnegie Mellon University in Pittsburgh, SRI International (Stanford Research Institute) at Menlo Park, California, and others at medical centers around the world are increasing the amount of knowledge and the applicability of these technologies. Some of the hurdles still to be overcome include accuracy validation, clinical evaluation, cost-benefit analysis, acceptance, regulatory issues, and liability.

In a broad sense, one of the best ways for clinicians to understand the applications and technologies discussed in this chapter is to create a general categorization of systems, such as passive, semi-active, and active, according to the level of independence given to computers or mechanical devices in performing actions.

1. *Passive.* Passive systems generally perform no action, but provide the surgeon with additional information prior to and during a procedure, augmenting the information provided by the real world. This category can be further broken down into the subcategories of surgical simulators, navigators, and aiming devices.

2. *Semiactive.* In semiactive systems "the surgical action is physically constrained to follow a predefined strategy. The action is guided, which means that the intervention is performed with respect to a previously defined strategy, but its final control depends on the surgeon."[1]

3. *Active.* Active systems are capable of performing isolated tasks, or entire procedures autonomously, under the watchful eye of the surgeon. A well-known example is the active system ROBODOC™. This system autonomously performs part of a total hip replacement surgery, creating the cavity for the femoral portion of the implant from a preoperative plan developed by a surgeon.

Although every system cannot be discussed here, an effort is made to choose representative systems in order to provide concrete examples. All systems discussed reflect the current state of technology and clinical applications.

III. PASSIVE SYSTEMS

SURGICAL SIMULATORS AND PREOPERATIVE PLANNERS

Surgical simulators and preoperative planners are passive systems that apply computational technologies formerly used in the aerospace industry for flight simulation and 3-D computer visualization techniques formerly used in CAD/CAM (computer-aided design/computer-aided manufacturing) to surgical practice. Standard imaging systems such as MR (magnetic resonance), CT (computed tomography), and others have long been used to create a series of individual medical images. Recent technological advances in both the hardware and software used in accessing medical images have allowed more sophisticated and accurate imaging systems to emerge. Although simulators and planners do not enter the surgical suite or perform a direct role in surgery, they provide valuable information and training to a surgeon prior to attempting a procedure. Using this data, a surgeon can develop a preoperative plan that defines how one or more tasks are to be performed during surgery. As passive systems, simulators and planners represent the least invasive form of computer assistance and make it possible for a surgeon to modify, optimize, and individualize an operative plan, thereby optimizing the clinical outcome. Surgical simulators also provide surgeons with an improved training ground for new, minimally invasive surgical procedures such as laparoscopic surgery, and they have the potential to improve surgical morbidity and mortality.[2]

EXAMPLE: TELEOS™   TELEOS™ is a unique software environment specifically developed to enhance surgical simulation technologies. TELEOS™ allows computational creation of physically based surgical fields and provides a real-time simulation environment. The software was written using C++ and GL and has been optimized to fully utilize the graphics performance of the Reality Engine Graphics supercomputer. Spline-based modeling is central to TELEOS™ and provides advantages such as ease in modeling anatomic movement and the ability to continuously vary details of cross sections that occur along a given spline, ensuring both optimal anatomic detail and real-time frame rates.[2] Computerized surgical simulations and virtual reality technologies are now being applied in training for new, minimally invasive surgical procedures such as laparoscopic surgery, which interposes a mechanical device between the surgeon's hands and the patient. The desired outcome of utilizing such technology in surgical training is to enhance patient contact during surgical procedures.

In order to create a "virtual organ" from medical imaging systems such as CT or MR, TELEOS™ first facilitates processing of registration and segmentation of sequential, two-dimensional data from these systems (Figure 7.1). Reconstructing 2-D images into basic 3-D objects requires accurate stacking and alignment of images. Tissue boundaries can be segmented at the same time as image registration to create outlines of the cross sections of each organ. A geo-

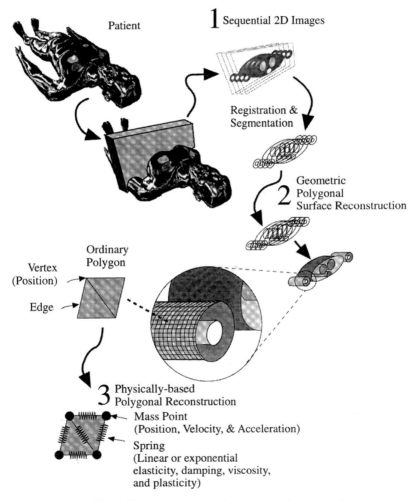

FIGURE 7.1. Modeling patient-specific anatomy for surgical simulation.

metric (polygonal) surface model is constructed in three dimensions once outlines (vectors) of all the cross sections of different tissues are available. In order to convert this geometric database into a physically based database, TELEOS™ simulates the behavior of tissues as flexible bodies based on mass elements and springs. Tissue characteristics can be configured by editing the physical parameters of the involved springs and mass points. [2]

Surgical simulations involving TELEOS™ include the "virtual abdomen" displayed at the 1994 annual meeting of the American Urological Association. A survey distributed to over 400 urologists at the meeting indicated an overwhelmingly positive response for the potential of virtual reality in surgical training.

NAVIGATORS

In image-guided surgery, preoperative medical data is used to plan, simulate, guide, or otherwise assist a surgeon in performing a medical procedure. Navigators provide the surgeon with a "road map" to structures more easily visualized by medical imaging techniques. Systems can be as simple as ultrasound guidance of a biopsy needle or as complex as superimposing the image of a tumor located by CT imaging onto a patient on the operating table.

EXAMPLE: IMAGE-GUIDED PEDICLE SCREW PLACEMENT   Currently several companies, including Medivision, Sofamor Danek, and Picker, have developed systems to meet the need for a reliable and safe method of pedicle screw insertion in spine surgery. Misplacement of pedicle screws inserted via conventional methods ranges between 6% and 40%.[3] Using the posterior approach to the spine during surgery allows only the exposure of the bony posterior elements, thus screws cannot be inserted completely with direct visual control. Navigation systems combine advanced stereotactic concepts and modern navigation techniques to control spinal surgical procedures through pre- and intraoperative planning and precise intraoperative guidance of pedicle screw insertion.[3] Presurgical spinal procedure planning begins with a good-quality preoperative CT image. CT data is later reconstructed into 2-D and 3-D views via segmentation, interpolation, and filter algorithms, in a manner similar to TELEOS™. Most systems can also utilize data from both tomographic images (MRI and CT) and projective images (X ray) as the basis for preoperative surgical planning.

The above image-guided systems address the traditional lack of direct links between image information, accessible anatomy, and the action of surgical instruments, by combining image-guided stereotaxis with advanced optoelectronic position-sensing techniques.[4] Various modules allow a surgeon preparing for a spinal operation to define the screw axes, to measure the depth of screw insertion and the diameter of the pedicles and to 'ride' along the chosen screw trajectory through the pedicle and the vertebral body. During the intraoperative phase of the process, the surgical tools are calibrated, and a dynamic reference base (DRB) is developed to establish a local reference coordinate system. A DRB clip is attached to the spinous process of one vertebra, thereby establishing a local reference system that provides information about the position of the vertebra in space. Next, anatomical landmarks on the bony surface of the posterior elements of the vertebra identified earlier are used in a paired point matching procedure that links the surgical object (vertebra) with the virtual object (tomographic image). These systems then transform the basic information, (i.e., the display of the tip of the tool on the computer screen) into navigational assistance or intraoperative real-time guidance and control of surgical procedures (Fig. 7.2).[4]

Before Medivision was introduced clinically, a thorough validation study was performed in Europe and a mathematical evaluation of the cascade of errors showed a mean deviation of 0.7 mm for any point displayed in the image from its real-world location. No complications occurred among six patients who underwent posterior fixation of degenerative lumbar spine segments using the system,

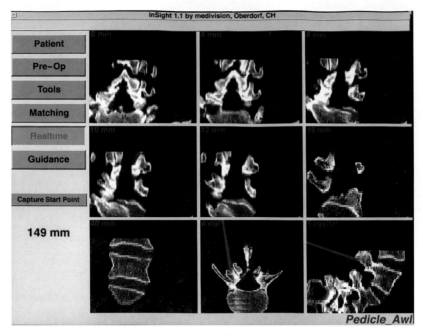

FIGURE 7.2. Real-time trajectory.

and a postoperative radiological evaluation confirmed accurate placement of the pedicle screws.[4] Nolte and Lund of the University of Bern indicate in several publications that the introductory phase of computer-assisted placement of pedicle screws in spine surgery indicates significant potential for future routine use and additional applications.

AIMING DEVICES

Aiming devices not only provide the surgeon with a map (as do navigators) but also a set of directions to follow to arrive at the desired destination. These systems usually assist the surgeon in performing some preoperatively planned task by guiding the surgeon's actions during the procedure.

EXAMPLE: HIPNAV   The Hip Navigation or HipNav system[5] is being developed jointly by Shadyside Hospital and Carnegie Mellon University to allow a surgeon to determine optimal, patient-specific acetabular implant placement and accurately achieve the desired placement during surgery. HipNav includes three components: a preoperative planner, a range of motion simulator, and an intraoperative tracking and guidance system.

The first step in using the HipNav system is the preoperative CT scan, which determines the patient's specific bony geometry. In the preoperative plan, the CT images allow the surgeon to determine appropriate implant size and placement.

Once the surgeon has selected the position of the acetabular implant, the range of motion simulator is used to determine the femoral positions (extension/flexion, abduction/adduction, and internal/external rotation) at which impingement would occur for that specific implant design and position. Based on this range of motion information, the surgeon may choose to modify the selected position in an attempt to achieve the "optimal" cup position for the specific patient.

The optimal patient specific plan is used by the HipNav system in the operating room on the day of surgery. HipNav permits the surgeon to determine where the pelvis and acetabulum are in operating room coordinates at all times during surgery. Knowledge of the position of the pelvis during all phases of surgery, and especially during preparation and implantation of the acetabular implant, permits the surgeon to accurately and precisely position the cup according to the preoperative plan.

There are several devices that are used intraoperatively to allow the surgeon to accurately execute the preoperative plan. One device is an Optotrak (Northern Digital, Ontario, Canada) optical tracking camera, which is capable of tracking the position of special light-emitting diodes (LEDs). In order to determine the location of the pelvis and the acetabular implant during surgery, Optotrak targets are attached to several conventional surgical tools (Fig. 7.3). The pelvis is tracked by attaching a target to the pelvic portion of a leg length caliper and inserting this device into the wing of the il-

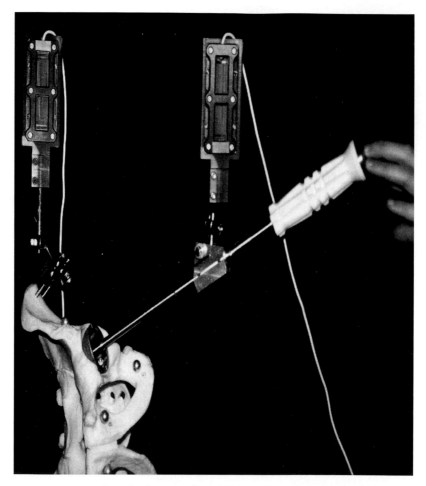

FIGURE 7.3. Standard surgical tools instrumented with optical tracking targets.

ium. The acetabular implant is tracked by attaching a second target to the handle of an acetabular cup holder and positioner. A third Optotrak target is required by the HipNav system to determine operating room coordinates (i.e., left, right, up, and down with respect to the surgeon).

Several key steps are necessary to use the HipNav intraoperative guidance system. One of the most important is the registration of preoperative information (i.e., the CT scan and preoperative plan) to the position of the patient on the operating room table. One limitation of current registration systems used in orthopedics is the need for pins to be surgically implanted into bone before preoperative images are acquired.

An alternative technique being used with HipNav is the use of surface geometry to perform registration. In this approach the surfaces of a bone (e.g., the pelvis or acetabulum) can be used to accurately align the intraoperative position of the patient to the preoperative plan without the use of pins or other invasive procedures. Using this technique, it is necessary to sense multiple points on the surface of the bone with a digitizing probe during surgery. These intraoperative data points are then matched to a geometric description of the bony surface of the patient derived from the CT images.

Once the location of the pelvis is determined via registration, navigational feedback can be provided to the surgeon on a television monitor. This feedback is used by the surgeon to accurately position the acetabular implant within the acetabular cavity. To accurately align the cup within the acetabulum in the position determined by the preoperative plan, the cross hairs representing the tip of the implant and the top of the handle must be aligned at the fixed cross hair in the center of the image (Fig. 7.4). Once aligned, the implant is in the preoperatively planned position and orientation.

Registration also allows the position of the pelvis to be tracked during surgery using the Optotrak system. This eliminates the need for rigid fixation of the pelvis. In addition, this tracking ability allows recording the position of the pelvis during surgery, and espe-

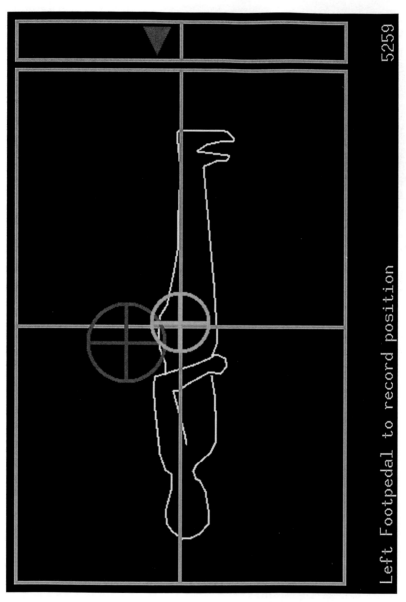

Left Footpedal to record position

FIGURE 7.4. Navigational feedback.

cially at key times such as at the time of implantation of the acetabular component or during range of motion testing.

The HipNav system holds the promise of reducing dislocation rates in primary and revision total hip replacement by optimizing the relative position of the acetabular implants and minimizing impingement. In addition, it will provide a new category of "smart" tools that will be useful to study issues in total hip replacement and ultimately other procedures. A cadaver trial was recently completed and human clinical trials of the HipNav system are underway at Shadyside Hospital as of April 1997.

IV. SEMIACTIVE SYSTEMS

EXAMPLE: AESOP AESOP (Automated Endoscopic System for Optimal Positioning) was developed to address the problems associated with a human assistant holding the endoscope in laparoscopic procedures.[6] Using a concept known as robotic enhancement technology (RET), AESOP is designed to compliment human manipulation in ways that traditional manufacturing or teleoperated robotic systems cannot. RET impacts all components of AESOP, including the mechanism, control system, and the man-machine interface. The result is a robotic system that teams with surgeons to perform tasks that exceed the capabilities of individual humans or machines.

Currently used in laproscopic procedures such as gall bladder removal, hernia repair, and laparoscopically assisted hysterectomy, AESOP is the first surgical robot to receive FDA approval, and has been involved in over 40 successful clinical trials at highly regarded institutions. The AESOP mechanism is a four-degree-of-freedom robot that clamps onto any standard surgical table. AESOP acts as a "third arm," allowing the surgeon to remain in complete control of the endoscope through a hand and/or foot controller interface. It can also store up to six endscope positions and return to them at the surgeon's command.

The key difference between an RET system like AESOP and more traditional robotic systems is the man-machine interface. Speech recognition technology and instrument-tracking interface architectures that could provide a more intuitive interface are currently being tested. To date, a speech interface has been implemented and tested, and image analysis algorithms have been validated in a non-real-time environment. Future work with AESOP is aimed at implementing image analysis and robot control algorithms in real-time in conjunction with completing the testing of the speech recognition technology. Such an interface would further expand the utility of the AESOP system by paving the way for a surgeon to control multiple robotic devices by a more seamless and intuitive interface.

V. ACTIVE SYSTEMS

In an active system some subtasks of the surgical strategy are performed with the help of an autonomous robotic system supervised by the surgeon and controlled by redundant sensors. Autonomous robots are active systems capable of performing individual tasks, or entire procedures autonomously (under the watchful eye of the surgeon). The best-known example of an active system is RO-BODOC™. This system autonomously creates the cavity for the femoral portion of a hip implant from a preoperative plan without need for direct control by the surgeon.

EXAMPLE: ROBODOC™ Addressing the shortcomings of the standard method of creating the femoral cavity for a hip implant, Integrated Surgical Systems, Inc. has developed a surgical robot, ROBODOC™, to create the cavity.

In 1993, 125,000 Americans underwent total hip arthroplasty,[7] a surgery to replace a damaged or diseased hip with an artificial implant. Cementless hip implant systems (a type often used on younger patients) rely on "natural" fixation from bone growing into the porous metal surfaces of the implant. Clinical and basic science research has shown that for ingrowth to occur, the cavity in the femur must be very exact such that any gap between bone and porous surface is less than 0.25 mm.

In the traditional method of performing hip replacement surgery, the surgeon selects the size of the implant by overlaying acetate templates over anterior/posterior and lateral X rays. This method yields only an approximate size of the implant and shows roughly where the implant should sit after its placement.

In the traditional surgical procedure for preparing the femur for a cementless implant, the surgeon uses a series of hand-held reamers and broaches (or chisels) to create the general size and shape of the cavity in bone. Although implant components are manufactured to a high level of precision, the method of creating the bone cavity has been much less precise. The reamers and broaches follow the canal of the bone and precise alignment is not always possible. In addition, these tools tend to bounce off hard cortical bone and tear away the softer trabecular bone, leaving large gaps that may result in improper ingrowth and early loosening of the implant.

ROBODOC™ addresses the problem of imprecise planning and cutting techniques by combining the tools of computer-aided design and an industrial robot to create a cavity precisely matched to the implant being placed. ROBODOC™ uses CT scan data to allow the surgeon to plan surgery in three dimensions on a computer workstation (ORTHODOC™).

The work plan created on ORTHODOC™ is converted to robot cutting instructions and transferred to the robot. During surgery the working end of the robot is a high-speed cutting burr that is guided by precise robotic movements to create a very accurately machined femoral cavity.

A ROBODOC™ procedure starts with surgical implantation of three small (4.0- and 6.5-mm) bone screws in the patient's greater

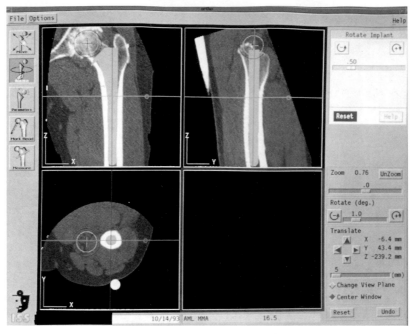

FIGURE 7.5. ORTHODOC™ preoperative planning.

trocanter and femoral condyles. These screws are used during the surgical procedure to orient the robot with the patient's leg at the time of surgery. A CT scan is then obtained taking special precautions to ensure that the patient does not move during the scan. The resulting CT data is transferred to the ORTHODOC™ presurgical workstation where it is preprocessed to detect any patient motion, derive the locations of the bone screws, and reconstructed into 3-D models. Once the preprocessing is complete, the surgeon selects and places an implant on the workstation. ORTHODOC™ allows the surgeon to precisely move and rotate the implant until the desired location is achieved. The result of this plan is used to create cutting instructions for the robot, and the cut plan is stored on tape.

During the surgery the pelvic portion of the implantation is performed in the normal fashion. When it is time for the femoral

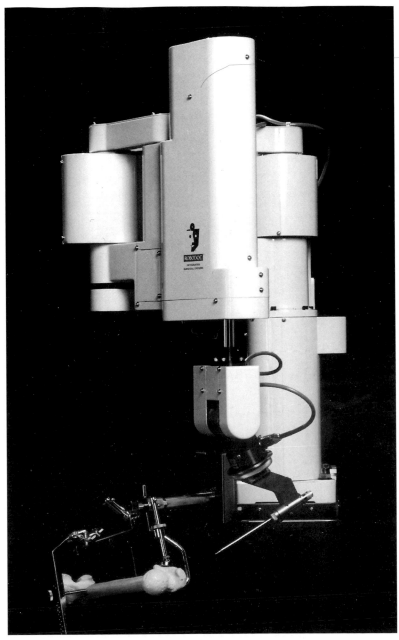

FIGURE 7.6. ROBODOC™ surgical robot and phantom femur.

cavity to be created, ROBODOC™ is moved into the surgical field and attached to the patient's femur with a fixator. Once the patient's femur is securely attached, the robot arm is guided to the center of each of the previously placed locator pins to orient the robot to the femur. ROBODOC™ calculates where the femur is with respect to its frame of reference and where the cutting path falls within that frame.

Once complete, the surgical team is directed to guide the cutting tool near the top of the femur and prepare for irrigation, (which cools the cutting tool and washes away debris). When the team is ready, the surgeon presses the start button on a hand-held control pendant. ROBODOC™ automatically cuts the cavity in the femur as was determined in the presurgical planning phase. Although the cutting is autonomous, the surgeon has the control to stop the robot via the hand-held pendant should something go wrong. Once the cutting is complete, ROBODOC™ is removed from the sterile field, the implant is placed, and the locator pins are removed. The surgery is completed in the usual fashion.

VI. CONCLUSION

Computer and robotic assistants are destined to enter mainstream medicine in the not so distant future. As with all new technology, it cannot automatically be assumed that these technologies will do the job better. Through scientifically based clinical trials, individual systems and applications must be evaluated to determine whether outcomes are improved and if the improvement in outcome is balanced against the higher costs of the new technology.

REFERENCES

1. Cinquin P, et al.: "Computer assisted medical interventions. *IEEE Eng Med Biol* (May/June 1995).

2. Merril JR, et al.: "Photorealistic interactive three-dimensional graphics in surgical simulation." In Morgan, K, et al. (eds.), Interactive Technology and the New Paradigm for Healthcare. Washington: IOS Press and Ohmsha, 1995:244–252.

3. Nolte LP, Müller M: "Computer assisted spine surgery."

4. Nolte LP: "A novel approach to computer assisted spine surgery."

5. DiGioia AM, HipNav: "Preoperative planning and intraoperative navigational guidance for acetabular implant placement in total hip replacement surgery."

6. Uecker DR, et al.: "A speech-directed multi-modal man-machine interface for robotically enhanced surgery." Proc First International Symposium on Medical Robotics and Computer Assisted Surgery, 1994.

7. American Academy of Orthopaedic Surgeons, http://www.aaos.org/wordhtml/press/hip_knee.htm.

TELEPRESENCE SURGERY

RICHARD M. SATAVA, M.D., F.A.C.S. AND
CDR. SHAUN B. JONES, M.D.

Telepresence surgery is being developed as a next generation of surgical technologies beyond laparoscopic surgery. We may discover in retrospect that laparoscopic surgery was principally a "transition" form of surgery on the way to telepresence surgery, much in the same way that the slide rule was a transition in computational mathematics from traditional mathematical "lookup tables" to the now ubiquitous electronic calculator. The word "telepresence" originates from the robotic and teleoperation engineering community and is most concisely defined by Thomas Sheridan as "the human operator receives sufficient information about the teleoperator and the task environment, displayed in a sufficiently natural way, that the operator feels physically present at the remote site."[1] Within the surgical area this would translate into a surgeon being at a central controlling console and receiving enough sensory input (sight, sound, touch) to feel as if the surgeon were actually directly performing surgery on the patient. Using these principles, telepresence surgery can offer two capabilities that are not possible

Cybersurgery: Advanced Technologies for Surgical Practice,
Edited by Richard M. Satava, M.D.
ISBN 0-471-15874-7   Copyright © 1998 by Wiley-Liss, Inc.

with current surgery: enhanced dexterity and remote access. Both of these capabilities are the result of recognizing the shortfalls of laparoscopic surgery and therefore attempting to make improvements. The purpose of dexterity enhancement is twofold: To return motion to the surgeon in such a manner that a difficult procedure has now a natural feeling, or to enhance the motion beyond limitations of human performance. In the former, laparoscopic surgery could be made to feel as natural as open surgery, with the computer interface translating the simple movements of open surgery to the awkward motions of laparoscopic surgery. With the latter it would mean giving accuracy, precision, position, or sensory input that is not currently possible by the unaided human hand, which is especially applicable in microsurgery and endovascular therapy. The issue of remote surgery for telepresence is actually an unintended consequence of using computers and other electronic systems to provide the dexterity enhancement. Once motion is converted into electronic signals by the computer, the possibility exists to transmit the signal to distant sites. The remote manipulator will perform the motion precisely as transmitted, whether it is a normal or enhanced action. Thus the telepresence surgery systems that were developed specifically to enhance the surgeons capabilities had the additional benefit of being fully capable of remote or telesurgery. The following examples of systems developed will elucidate both the value of dexterity enhancement and remote access.

Laparoscopic surgery suddenly emerged onto the surgical scene and immediately gained acceptance in spite of the limitations imposed on the skill of the surgeon. Gone are natural stereoscopic vision, dexterity, and the sense of touch. With laparoscopy, for the first time surgeons began to use the information equivalent of vision (the video monitor) and use instruments for which they could not directly see the tips (except in the video monitor). Thus laparoscopic surgery has more in common with "teleoperation" (or more specifically "telepresence surgery") than conventional "open" surgery. Teleoperation uses sensors to detect hand motion, convert the motion to electronic signals (information), transmit to a remote location, and then exactly reproduce the motions. Likewise laparoscopic surgery uses instruments in which the surgeon uses hand motion to direct the movement of the tip of an instrument in a remote location (inside the abdomen) that cannot be directly visualized. If one considers laparoscopic surgery as a very primitive form of teleoperation, then telepresence surgery (remote surgery between distant cities or places) is the next logical development. In one sense the surgeon's hand motions can be considered as just one more form of information—it is no longer blood and guts, it is bits and bytes. When telesurgery achieves its full potential in both dexterity enhancement and remote delivery of care, it could replace much of laparoscopic surgery, leaving those procedures that are optimal for the laparoscopic approach to continue in their specific small niche.

The time could not be more perfect. We now have the right type of surgeon to take advantage of this new information age technology. First it was the "Nintendo Surgeon" for laparoscopic surgery; now it is the "Digital Physician". Older-generation surgeons have difficulty with laparoscopic surgery because they have been trained to operate with a single hand-to-eye axis—from the eye through the hand to the object to be manipulated. Just as a child manipulates toys in a sandbox, this same single direct hand-eye axis is used for all daily actions, from eating our meals to operating on patients. However, since the integration of video technology into the daily life of our children, there is an emergence of a younger generation that has trained on video games and developed multiple hand-eye axes. They can be looking at a video monitor in one direction while accurately controlling a computer joystick in a totally different direction. They are capable of decoupling the oculo-vestibular axis for visual orientation from their haptic-proprioceptive axis for manipulation. Because this decoupling is one of the major factors that make laparoscopic surgery difficult, they have an intuitive, natural ability with these new hand-eye skills, just as children who learn a language are able to speak it with all the intuitiveness and accents of a native, whereas adults may be precise in their use of the language but never be able to speak with the native naturalness. Thus our younger surgeons who have grown up in the video/electronic generation are not only comfortable with the new technology, but they are demanding it. They play video games, "surf" over Internet and the "information super highway," or become educated with computer-aided instruction, multimedia, and virtual reality. To them the future is Now, and it is all digital.

Having understood the potential to improve upon laparoscopic surgery, which is provided by using the power of digital information in the form of telepresence, Green et al. developed a system that would return to the surgeon the 3-D vision, dexterity, and sense of touch that was lost during laparoscopic surgery.[2, 3] The system created is called *telepresence surgery*; it was initially designed to enhance the dexterity of the surgeon to a point where laparoscopic surgery felt as if it was being performed as open surgery (Fig. 8.1).

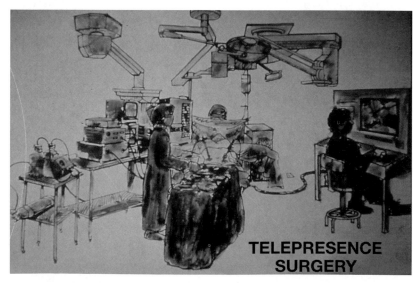

FIGURE 8.1. Telepresence surgery, original concept: The surgeon sits next to the patient and operates from the surgical workstation to regain 3-D vision, dexterity, and sense of touch.

At the surgeon console (Fig. 8.2), by holding instrument handles that look and feel like actual surgical instruments (Fig. 8.3), the surgeon looks down into a 3-D image that appears like open surgery with the instrument tips and abdominal organs easily viewed directly in front. When the handles move, the tips move and feel the resistance of the tissues; only there is nothing at the surgical console. Instead there is a remote manipulator (tele-manipulator) adjacent to the surgeon that is actually performing the surgery (Fig.

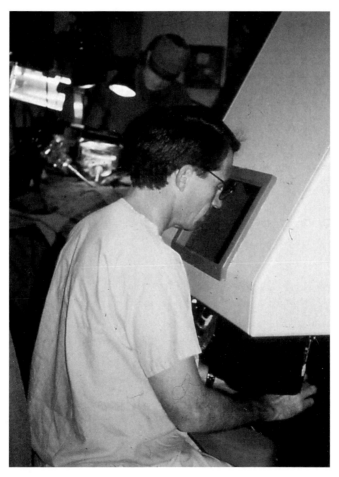

FIGURE 8.2. The Green telepresence surgery system: The surgeon at the "surgical console" (courtesy of Dr. Phil Green, SRI International, Menlo Park, CA).

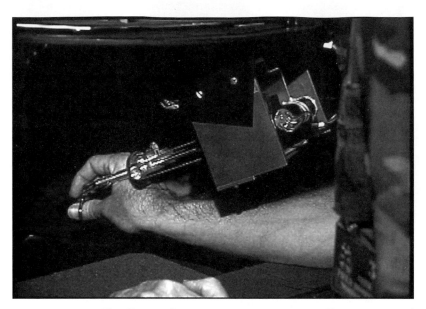

FIGURE 8.3. The Green telepresence surgery system : Close up view of the surgical handles on the "surgical console" (courtesy of Dr. Phil Green, SRI International, Menlo Park, CA).

8.4). Thus the perception of doing open surgery is now returned to the surgeon. However, it was not until the system had begun animal trials that it became apparent that the surgeon did not have to be in the same room, or even city or country. The surgical console is electronically attached to the manipulator site by nothing more than a wire, so a system designed for dexterity enhancement has the additional advantage of being a system capable of remote surgery. The second-generation system is now completed as the SRI Telesurgical System; it has increased range of motion to approximate natural human work capability and advanced telecommunications that specifically address the remote capabilities. The current system is not designed to provide capabilities beyond natural motion. Initial animal studies have been completed and reported by Bowersox,[4] demonstrating the capability to perform numerous common surgical procedures (Table 8.1). The remote manipulators of the Green-SRI

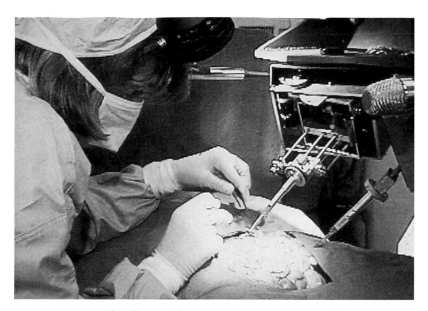

FIGURE 8.4. The Green telepresence surgery system: The remote robotic surgical instruments, which are being controlled by the surgeon from the console and assisted by the nurse at the remote site, here performed on pig intestines (courtesy of Dr. Phil Green, SRI International, Menlo Park, CA).

TABLE 8.1. PROCEDURES
DEMONSTRATED FOR TELESURGERY

Gastrostomy and closure
Gastric resection
Bowel anastomosis
Liver laceration suture
Liver lobe resection
Splenectomy
Aortic graft replacement
Arteriotomy repair

telesurgery system have been mounted inside an experimental military armored operating room vehicle and surgical procedures on animals have been demonstrated over a 5-km wireless transmission between a MASH tent and the remote vehicle.[5]

There are two other current systems under similar development. Professors Gehard Buess and Herman Rininsland of the Forschungszentrum of Karlsruhe, Germany,[6] have developed the ARTEMIS system (Fig. 8.5), which has a remote telemanipulator system that is controlled from a surgical console with the input devices behind the surgeon so that the master controllers are "reaching over" surgeon, much the way in which a golf instructor stands behind and holds a golf club together with a student. This permits master control in a very natural fashion, including tracking the forearm and shoulder motions as well as the hand motions. In front of the surgeon is a bank of large monitors of the operative site as well as a panoramic view of the operating room. Thus there is a very large work space directly in front of the monitors for the master controllers to work. Rather than feeling as if the surgeon is out-

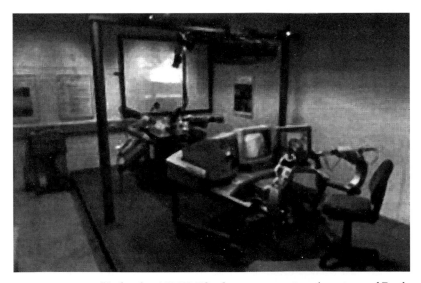

FIGURE 8.5. Karlsruhe ARTEMIS telesurgery system (courtesy of Profs. Gehard Buess and Herman Rininsland, Forschungszentrum, Karlsruhe).

side the patient and operating down into the abdomen, the system almost gives the perception that the surgeon is holding the tips of the instruments while inside of the abdomen. The system of Profs. Russell Taylor and Wolfgang Daum have remote manipulators similar to the Karlsruhe system; however, one of the master controllers is a glove that controls a three-fingered hand to grasp and manipulate tissue.

In the area of dexterity enhancement, there are a number of systems that are being developed to extend the capabilities beyond human performance. Professor Ian Hunter of the Massachusetts Institute of Technology[7] is developing such a system for ophthamological surgery (Fig. 8.6). For laser retinal surgery, a precision of at least 25 μ is required because of the close spacing of the retinal vessels. Should a vessel be struck, a retinal hematoma could occur with subsequent blindness. The unassisted human hand is not capable of positioning with an accuracy of greater than 200 μ. In addition muscle fatigue rapidly induces an intention tremor, at a frequency of 8–14 Hz (cycles

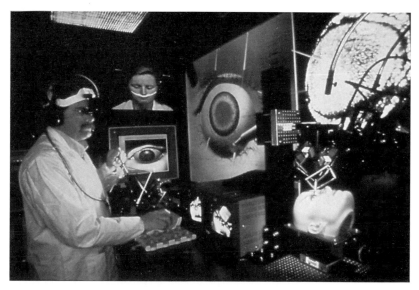

FIGURE 8.6. Enhanced dexterity system for ophthamology (courtesy of Dr. Ian Hunter, MIT, Cambridge).

per second). To complicate matters, the eye has a natural saccade motion of 200 Hz. The Hunter telepresence system tracks the motion of the eye and is designed to scale the motion of the hand up by a hundredfold, so 1 cm of the surgeon's hand motion moves the laser 10 μ. The video image magnifies the retinal vessels to the size of a finger. By applying sophisticated digital signal processing (DSP) and signal filtering techniques through the computer interface, the normal tremor of the human hand can be removed. Combining all of these techniques permits accuracy and precision to 10 μ, which is greater than an order magnitude more accurate than the unaided hand.

There continues to be development in the area of the end effectors, which are the "instruments" that are at the ends of the remote telemanipulator. The two issues that must be addressed are (1) the dexterity, force and precision of the manipulation, and (2) the quality of sensory input returned to the surgeons' hands. A number of innovative end effectors are being investigated. One is the Daum Hand (Fig. 8.7) by Wolfgang Daum of Germany which has a dexter-

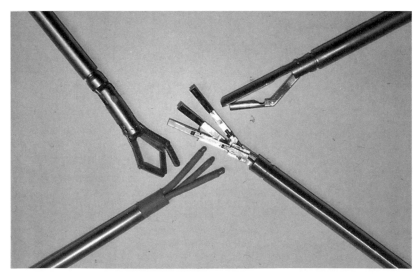

FIGURE 8.7. Dexterous three-fingered miniature "hand" (courtesy of Wolfgang Daum, Daum Inc., Baltimore, MD).

ous three-fingered miniature "hand" or grasper that is controlled by a glovelike device that provides both control and a simple level of sensory response. Other investigators such as Alfred Cuschieri of Dundee Scotland and Ranjan Mukerjee of Michigan State University are investigating shape memory alloy materials to increase the dexterity of the end effectors. Numerous investigators, including Gehard Buess and David Brock of the Massachussetts Institute of Technology (MIT), are embedding miniature tactile devices into the tips of the graspers to add the sense of touch to the force-reflection feedback that provides the sense of pressure in the current-generation instruments.

All the systems are being developed using direct connection by electronic cable between the master and slave units, or over very short wireless communication links. Ultimately the goal will be to provide remote expert surgical capabilities worldwide, and perhaps with a specific focus to third world countries where the surgical and procedural capabilities do not exist. Under any long distance transmission it is likely that satellite communication will be used. Since the geosynchronous satellites are approximately 22,000 mi above the earth, the time to send and receive the signals is greater than 1.5 s (1500 mss). This technical barrier is referred to as the "delay," "latency," or "lag" problem. The importance to the latency is that the human operator is not able to compensate for significant transmission delays. For example, we know from data on astronaut training, a delay between the hand motion and the movement of the space shuttle arm of greater than 25 ms is not perceptible. At 50 ms the operator knows that there is something "wrong" (something does not feel right, though it is not clear what it is) but automatically and intuitively compensates. By 100 ms of latency, the delay is obvious, but the operator can be trained to accommodate the delay. However, at 200 ms, it is nearly impossible to compensate, even with extensive training. In addition the telesurgical systems, which have closed-loop feedback for the sense of touch, become unstable when delays of greater than 200 ms are introduced. Therefore in the immediate future it is anticipated that the telesurgical systems will only be used in situations where the technical barrier of delay is less than 200 ms, which includes wireless transmission of 50 km or less, or over networks of 200 mi or less.

In addition to their use for patient care, telesurgery systems can be used for surgical simulation. Because all telesurgery systems have a monitor or other display to provide the image at the remote site, this image can be replaced by a computer-generated image. Now the broad spectrum of surgical care can be provided through the same system. If the image is a model of normal anatomy derived from a standard source such as the Visible Human, teaching in anatomy or pathology, or training on a specific procedure, can be done. However, if the model is generated from patient-specific data, such as MRI, CT, or ultrasound, the system can be used to do preoperative planning or even rehearsal of the surgical procedure to be performed on that specific patient the next day, permitting the optimal procedure from many possible choices for that patient. Theoretically, on the day of surgery, while the anesthesiologist is putting the patient to sleep, the surgeon could practice the intended surgical procedure on the patient-specific model, and after the patient is anesthetized, the surgeon can "flip a switch" and continue to operate, but now on the patient rather than the model of the patient.

The clinical implementation of these technologies is more of a challenge than the scientific path to their technical development. The problem of latency has been addressed above; other scientific challenges include optimizing the safety of the systems, improving the reliability of the precision and control, increasing both dexterity and sensory input, miniaturizing the current size of systems to be less bulky and intrusive in the operating theater, ensuring a robust telecommunication transmission and developing manufacturing and commercialization to reduce the overall costs of the systems.

While we understand and quantify where the technical barriers are and can scientifically approach some solutions, it is less clear how to solve the nontechnical barriers to clinical implementation.

These barriers include legal, regulatory, financial, and behavioral. When a telesurgical procedure is performed, under whose authority and responsibility is the granting of privileges, certification, and quality assurance—the central institution where the surgeon is located, or the remote location where the patient and less trained health care professional (general surgeon, general practitioner, physician extender) is located? Who is "responsible" for the patient, the surgeon back at the medical center doing the procedure or the family practitioner who has been managing the patient and is present at the patient's side during the procedure? Are we creating a new generation of itinerant surgeons—the "tele-itinerant surgeon"? Should a mishap occur, under whose legal authority is the case determined, especially if the surgeon and patient are in different states or countries? Also under which state's regulations are the implementation of the telesurgery controlled? As in much of telemedicine today, reimbursement is not allowed without "face to face" contact between patient and doctor; thus who will perform telesurgery if there is no reimbursement and at the same time be exposed to all the legal liability? But probably the most important facet is the issue of behavior and acceptance, both on the part of the physician as well as the patient.

Telesurgery faces the behavioral issues of both the surgeons' reluctance to have a "robot" interposed between them and their patient, as well as the patients' perception of being operated on by a robot. However, there are three distinct situations where telesurgery will be of value, despite the resistance to behavioral change. The first is where the alternative to telesurgery is no surgery and perhaps certain death. Second is the fact that as the technology of telepresence increases, the illusion permits a near-realistic perception of being at the remote area, which can promote and perhaps even enhance the feeling of actually "being there." The third is the most important, which is as our new generation of surgeons emerge, the use of telesurgery will be accepted as fact and will be embraced as the standard method for surgery. Likewise a younger and more sophisticated patient population will expect the use of computer-enhanced and remote surgery as a manifestation of high-quality health care.

While the acceptance of telesurgery depends on the complex mix of social and technical factors, it will remain the sole responsibility of the surgeon to guarantee that the ethical and moral issues of the new technologies will be upheld and that any new technology will be used individually with compassion and caring for each and every individual patient.

REFERENCES

1. Sheridan TB: "Defining our terms." *Presence* (1992) 1:272–74.
2. Green PS, Satava RM, Hill JR, Simon IB: "Telepresence: Advanced tele-operator technology for minimally invasive surgery" (Abstr). *Surg Endosc* (1992) 6:90.
3. Hill JR, Green PS, Jensen JF, Gorfu Y, Shah AS: "Telepresence surgery demonstration system." *Proc IEEE Internat Conf on Robotics and Automation* (1994) 4:2302–2307.
4. Bowersox JC, Shah A, Jensen J, Hill J, Cordts PR, Green PS: "Vascular applications of telepresence surgery: Initial feasibility studies in swine." *J Vasc Surg* (1996) 23:281–7.
5. Satava RM: "Advanced technology for battlefield medicine." In Laires MF, Ladeira MF, Christensen JP (eds.), *Health in the New Communications Age.* Washington: IOS Press and Ohmsha. 1995:38–40.
6. Buess and Rhinsland: The ARTEMIS system. Site visit at the Forschungzentrum, Karlsruhe, Germany, May 1996.
7. Hunter IW, Doukoglou TD, Lafontaine SR, et al.: "A teleoperated micro-surgical robot and associated virtual environment for eye surgery." *Presence* (1993) 4:265–80.
8. Spitzer VM, Whitlock DG: "Electronic imaging of the human body. Data storage and interchange format standards." In Vannier MW, Yates RE, Whitestone JJ (eds.), *Proc Electronic Imaging of the Human Body Working Group,* March 9–11, 1992:66–68.

TELEMEDICINE, TELEMENTORING, AND TELEPROCTORING

CDR. SHAUN B. JONES, M.D. AND RICHARD M. SATAVA, M.D., F.A.C.S.

Changes in society—whether demographic or economic—usually mandate changes in the social services. Indeed, faced with such pervasive challenges as an aging population, burgeoning medical technologies, rising costs, and diminishing federal subsidies, health care providers throughout the Western world are confronting inevitable—and urgent—reforms.

Increasingly physicians are finding that traditional methods of health care delivery are fast becoming obsolete. As society prepares to enter the twenty-first century, it must come to grips with the stark reality that the ability of health care providers to diagnose and treat illnesses far outdistances their capacity to deliver top-quality care to large segments of the population. Medicine today has become a highly complex, costly, and diversified discipline, and it promises to become even more so during the coming decades.

Cybersurgery: Advanced Technologies for Surgical Practice,
Edited by Richard M. Satava, M.D.
ISBN 0-471-15874-7   Copyright © 1998 by Wiley-Liss, Inc.

"As a result of geographic and socioeconomic barriers, more than 40 million people in the U.S. are disenfranchised from our health-care system," says Jay H. Sanders, president of the American Telemedicine Association in Washington, DC. "Even more frustrating is the realization that while our skill at diagnosing and treating disease continues to improve, our ability to distribute and deliver that care has not."

Yet today's physicians and surgeons can now call upon the growing resources of "telemedicine" (a medical consultation carried out at a distance) or "telesurgery" (an operation performed at a distance). By way of advanced computational techniques, they may even be able to perform an "augmented" or "enhanced" procedure, whose precision is increased by technology, as in microsurgery or computer-aided implants.

So many and varied are the kinds of telecommunications and computing systems now used in medicine that the term "telemedicine" has become an umbrella covering many applications. According to the National Institute of Medicine's 1996 Telemedicine report,[1] "for more than 30 years, clinicians, health services researchers, and others have been investigating the use of advanced telecommunications and computer technologies to improve health care. At the intersection of many of these efforts is telemedicine—a combination of mainstream and innovative information technologies." To include as many activities as possible under this umbrella term, the Institute of Medicine defines *telemedicine* as "the use of electronic information and communications technologies to provide and support health care when distance separates the participants." The critical features of all telemedical procedures is that they seek to bridge the distance between doctor and patient.

Applications of the new technologies appear primarily in the following areas:

Medicine. Diagnosing, treating, and monitoring patients at a distance (telemedicine); informing patients; fostering preventive care; relaying patient information through improved displays and models.

Surgery. Enhancing, planning, and simulating procedures to prepare for surgery; performing surgical procedures at a distance (telesurgery).

Training. Teaching, monitoring, and proctoring at a distance; practicing skills through simulations; (tele-mentoring).

Education. Transmitting information to patients, physicians, and students; conveying technical information through displays and models; rehabilitating patients (tele-education or distant learning).

Research and development. Visualizing massive medical databases; modeling systems; designing new tools, instruments, procedures, and workspaces; testing new equipment and ideas (virtual collaboration).

Some specialty areas have already arisen within telemedicine and telesurgery. They include telepathology, teleradiology, telementoring, and teleproctoring. Each specialty offers distinct features.

Telepathology, for example, involves a pathologist examining specimens, either visible or microscopic, using a digital image presented on a video monitor. Such techniques have proved effective for primary and secondary diagnoses and for quality assurance.

Teleradiology, one of the fastest-growing specialty areas, permits radiologists in different medical centers to review digital images of scans or films without having to rely on the awkward, time-consuming transport of film jackets. For example, a CT scan that incorporates 50 images, if properly compressed into a 25 megabyte file, will transmit over a dedicated digital line (e.g., a T1 fiber-optic connection) in a mere 16.5 s—enhancing timely diagnoses and patient treatment.

Telementoring and teleproctoring, in a similar vein, involve an experienced physician or surgeon guiding a trainee during an actual procedure, performed and monitored from a distance. Derived from the name of the teacher of Odysseus, the term "mentor" refers to a wise and faithful counselor. Thus a telementor serves his trainee by offering experience, advice, or direction during procedural training, including surgery.

I. TELEMEDICINE: DIAGNOSES AND PATIENT MONITORING

Advanced information and telecommunication systems have brought benefits to the traditional medical problems of diagnosing and treating illnesses in emergency or difficult situations. Delivering highly specialized medical care to patients in remote areas of the United States and developing countries presents no less a need or challenge than does delivering such care to soldiers on a battlefield.

"One of the major barriers to health care for patients in isolated or impoverished communities is the inadequate number of physicians who choose to establish or maintain their practices outside of a major metropolitan area," observes Sanders. Moreover "transportation costs also increase as patients must be transferred to distant hospitals. These transfers are deleterious not only to the patient but also to the community as well. As a local hospital's bed census declines, its fiscal viability, along with the socio-economic fabric of the community, is threatened.[2]"

In one response to this perceived need, the Medical College of Georgia (MCG) instituted a telemedicine system in 1991. By way of interactive voice and color video telecommunications with biomedical telemetry, physicians at the system's "hub" in Augusta examine and treat patients in rural hospitals, ambulatory health centers, nursing homes, emergency rooms, correctional institutions, and international health facilities. Patients receive top-rate care locally, without expensive and distressing travel to a faraway medical center.

In trauma cases this electronic expertise has helped reduce morbidity and mortality. Physicians can obtain patient history, conduct a physical exam, and transfer information back and forth as if the patient were in a neighboring office. Zoom-focus cameras, electronic stethoscopes, EKGs, and echocardiograms enable physicians ranging from cardiologists to dermatologists to perform detailed exams. For example, using remote technology, ophthalmologists can view retinas, otorhinolaryngologists can monitor laryngoscopies, and gastroenterologists can navigate endoscopes. Moreover radiologists can interpret X rays and scans, pathologists can scrutinize tissue samples, and gynecologists can guide laparoscopes.[2]

A computer-controlled switching matrix enables MCG's physicians to network telemedically between the university's medical center and multiple satellite locations. Video consultations can be recorded and archived for quality assurance and teaching purposes. Patient records, prescriptions, consultations notes, and medical data can all be swiftly sent by fax or modem. During a procedure images can be "frozen" and stored, printed, or transferred for analysis. A special electronic pen permits physicians to annotate X rays, EKGs, and MRIs. A physician can simultaneously view and compare a live patient with an X ray or a scan.

To help monitor and treat "revolving-door" hospital patients with chronic conditions, MCG physicians have installed interactive video and medical diagnostic equipment in patients' homes. The MCG telemedicine network now includes 59 Georgia hospitals and clinics. Of patients who might have required transfer from rural hospitals to specialized care facilities, 86% can today remain where they are. As a result of this pilot program, says Sanders, "the impact of the Telemedicine System has been so significant in the Augusta region that the Medical College of Georgia is proposing to the Governor that it be replicated statewide."[3]

According to figures cited in the Global Telemedicine Report,[4] 48 of 50 U.S. states have telemedicine centers, and the remaining two states have remote referral sites. To serve developing countries, organizations such as the Cleveland Clinic Foundation, and the Mayo Clinic, Rochester are exploring systems to provide consultations abroad.

At Carnegie Mellon University in Pittsburgh, researchers have hooked laptop computers into a wireless communications system, enabling nurses to receive doctors' orders, chart patients' progress, consult medical references, and even use educational videos when caring for patients in their homes.[5]

At the University of Minnesota, Minneapolis, Dr. Stanley M. Finkelstein has studied the benefits of advanced technology for lung transplant patients. Following surgery, patients test themselves daily at home, record results automatically, and transmit them to a database and their physician. The system increases the rate of testing, lowers the cost, and detects problems before symptoms appear.[3]

Technology now permits the home-monitoring of newborns with cord-entanglement problems. Once mothers have returned home following delivery, they can set up infant monitoring equipment, hooked remotely to a physician's computer, that follows the baby's heart rate in an effort to preempt trouble.[6]

The University of Kansas has operated a telemedicine program since 1991, when Kansas University Medical Center in Kansas City hooked up electronically to the Area Health Education Center in Hays, Kansas. Given the state's low-density population—only 2.4 physicians per 1000 residents statewide, with 82 of 105 counties having fewer than 1 physician per 1000 residents—rural medical treatment remains critical.

Today 13 medical facilities throughout Kansas communicate digitally, with an additional 6 rural sites under development. A "one-stop" telemedicine service provides impromptu consultations, locates specialists, and schedules appointments and laboratory tests. Specialty clinics exist online for remote consults in oncology, psychiatry, infectious diseases, pulmonary disorders, hematology, and cardiology.

A variety of education programs for patients and physicians take place telemedically, ranging from diabetes to Parkinson's disease. A special "teleoncology" practice has been established: By way of high-resolution color video cameras and monitors, connected by a dedicated digital line, oncologists converse with patients and perform examinations. In similar fashion a "virtual clinic" diagnoses and treats rural patients with Parkinson's disease, the majority of whom might never receive treatment at all.

Following a similar model, a "tumor board" meeting of oncologists, pathologists, and radiologists takes place each month between the Carolinas Medical Center in Charlotte, NC, and the Watauga Medical Center in Boone, NC. At these meetings specialists review difficult cases with the 30 surgeons, chemotherapists, and health-support workers at Watauga's Cancer Center from a specially equipped telemedicine room in Charlotte.[7]

To serve rural areas of North Carolina, the East Carolina University (ECU) School of Medicine in Greenville has established a telemedicine network. Between August 1992 and September 1996, ECU physicians from 29 specialties conducted 1011 telemedical consultations, 55% of which involved dermatology. Typically a nurse at a rural clinic or prison "spoke site" presents a patient to a "hub site" physician, who examines the patient from a sound-proof booth rigged with telediagnostic tools (i.e., stethoscope, otoscope, opthalmascope, and dermatology camera). Currently the telemedical network includes a hub at the ECU Medical School and spoke sites at 4 rural hospitals, 2 clinics, 1 naval hospital, and 1 maximum-security prison. For emergency care, a hub emergency care department provides links to rural hospital emergency rooms.[8]

Telemedicine has great potential for treating inmates in prisons. A network of 31 ECU physicians from 15 disciplines are performing telemedical consultations with patients at North Carolina's maximum-security Central Prison in Raleigh. Physicians interview the patients by way of a telemedicine link, diagnose illnesses, and prescribe medications. They may even examine patients using digital stethoscopes and a hand-held dermatology camera. Telemedical consultations have cut the $700 cost of transporting a prisoner for medical services and reduced the risk of escape.[8] Similarly physicians at the University of Texas, Medical Branch at Galveston, treat 45 to 65 cases each week using a telemedical link to the local prison.[9] In Colorado, corrections officials are evaluating the use of telemedicine for treating prisoners.

For telepsychiatry, the Eastern Oregon Human Services Consortium (EOHSC) has organized a program called the Rural Options for Development and Educational Opportunities (RODEO) NET, which connects mental health programs in 13 eastern Oregon counties. So far the program provides case consultations, patient evaluation, medication management, and crisis response through a 24-hour emergency service.[1]

To monitor patients postsurgically in a nursing home, physicians at the Stanford University Medical Center and neighboring Lytton Garden Health Care Center established a telemedical link to supervise health care for low-income senior citizens. Using an interactive video link, surgeons receive notes from physicians at the nursing home, then examine patients in a specially equipped room. Dermatology and psychiatry consultations have also proved practical. Physicians and surgeons at Stanford and the National Institutes of Health are collaborating to develop a telemedicine system through which they can monitor patients in the intensive care unit, at a distance, using the internet.

Other examples of regional telemedicine projects include the Iowa Communications Network, a fiber-optic system linking Iowa's 3 main medical centers, has held 10 pathology, 10 cardiology, 100 echocardiography teleconsultations, plus 250 noninvasive vascular imaging transmissions.[10] The Eastern Montana Telemedicine Network, during the first year of its videoconferencing pilot, permitted rural health care providers to treat successfully 95% of their patients who needed distant specialists.[3] The Cleveland Memorial Hospital in Shelby, NC, has used telemedicine to improve the efficiency of its trauma center. The Oklahoma Telemedicine Network, which connects 45 rural hospitals in the state, transfers patient reports and slides to aid patient care.[3] The High Plains Rural Health Network is expanding services to cover the frontier areas, which have fewer than six inhabitants per square mile, of northeastern Colorado, northwest Kansas, and southwest Nebraska.[11]

So concerned about—and committed to—the progress of telemedicine for reaching and treating patients in rural areas are public health officials that in 1995 the Western Governor's Association, representing 22 U.S. states and territories, convened a Telemedicine Policy Review Group, consisting of telemedicine experts and senior health officials. The group prepared a series of background papers on barriers to telemedicine and put forth recommendations to help overcome them and implement a program to serve the public.

While stating that "today, telemedicine holds more potential than ever to fulfill its promise of improved access to health care for under served rural citizens," the panel concluded that "previous high costs and technical limitations on telemedicine technology have been significantly reduced and are no longer a primary barrier." Rather, the panelists concluded that the most significant barriers to telemedicine stem from inadequate information infrastructure and uncoordinated infrastructure planning; regulatory distortions, limitations on competition, and fragmented demand; public and private reimbursement policies that do not compensate for telemedicine services; physician licensing and credentialing rules that discourage physicians from practicing telemedicine within states and across state lines; concerns about malpractice liability associated with telemedicine; and, concerns about the confidentiality of patient information.[12]

The Governor's Report went on to outline some potential legal and administrative measures that health officials can take to try to overcome these obstacles and foster the growth of telemedical patient care.

Historically, telemedicine has come a long way since *Radio News* first published an article in its April 1924 issue speculating about a "radio doctor" linked to a patient electronically via sound and picture. But the first known reference to telemedicine in the medical literature appeared in 1950, describing telephone transmission of radiology images in Pennsylvania between West Chester and Philadelphia. Based on this system, radiologists at Montreal's Jean-Talon Hospital in Canada designed a simple teleradiology network.[1]

In 1959 University of Nebraska physicians began using interactive television to transmit neurological examinations to students across campus. And in 1964 clinicians at the Nebraska Psychiatric Institute in Omaha began using a microwave link with the Norfolk State Hospital 112 miles away for consultations, including neurological examinations, speech therapy, difficult diagnoses, and group therapy.[1]

During the 1960s and 1970s several U.S. hospitals—including Massachusetts General Hospital in Boston and Mt. Sinai School of Medicine in New York City—experimented with limited telemedical links. An unusual partnership among the U.S. Indian Health Service, NASA, and the Lockheed Company led to project STARPAHC (Space Technology Applied to Rural Papago Advanced Health Care), which experimentally provided medical services via satellite to astronauts and residents of a rural reservation.[1]

Today more than 60 telemedicine programs throughout the United States have set up facilities capable of using interactive television for treating patients. In the case of teleradiology, in 1994 alone 15 teleradiology programs in North America serviced 90 remote sites and interpreted approximately 22,000 images. An estimated 60 telepathology systems are currently in use in the United States.[13]

II. TELEMENTORING AND TELEPROCTORING

Telemedicine can serve to train, proctor, and certify less experienced surgeons. An expert surgeon in a central location, connected electronically with a less experienced surgeon at a remote site, can effectively guide, consult, proctor, and ultimately certify the trainee.

Tremendous progress has taken place since Dr. Michael DeBakey first demonstrated the concept of telementoring on May 2, 1965. At Houston's Methodist Hospital, DeBakey replaced an aortic valve in a patient, transmitting live audio and video of the operation to the Geneva University Medical Center in Switzerland. This process enabled surgeons to see, hear, and follow the procedure in real time across the Atlantic Ocean.[14]

In telementoring, an experienced surgeon remotely educates and trains a surgical student or less experienced practitioner in specific skills. In teleproctoring, the skilled surgeon remotely evaluates and certifies a surgical trainee or resident. The differences between the roles played by preceptors and proctors have led to considerable confusion in the medical community when questions of authority and responsibility arise. While a preceptor actively participates in the learning and teaching process, a proctor only evaluates procedures impartially and reports on his observations. This distinction has proved critical in sorting out some of the dilemmas, particularly when it comes to determining liability during a telesurgical procedure.

Early investigations into telementoring and teleproctoring have been performed by Rosser, Payne, et al.[14] and by Talamini, Cubano, et al. Rosser, based in Yale Medical Center in New Haven, has telementored students in such far-flung locations as Honolulu, Hawaii, and The Netherlands.[15] Kavoussi, et al.,[16] based at the Johns Hopkins Medical Center in Baltimore, has teleproctored laparoscopic hernia repairs on a U.S. Navy ship in the Pacific Ocean. Dr. Peter Go,[15] stationed in Belgium, has teleproctored laparoscopic hiatus hernia repair operations in Nieuwegein, The Netherlands. Maresceaux et al.[17] are teaching students remotely from their base at the University of Strasbourg.

As a result of these new technologies, many important issues arise regarding the training, certification, and practice of remote surgery. On the one hand, surgeons must consider technical complications: What if a communications link becomes interrupted, electrical power fails, or a computer suffers a "glitch?" On the other hand, legal questions too appear: Does a physician need two licenses to practice medicine remotely across state lines or between countries? In the event of errors or complications, which state laws are followed? Who must be held responsible if the primary surgeon is unable to respond to a patient crisis?

From the perspective of surgical education, one wonders: If a teacher or proctor is not physically present during an operation, will the quality of instruction and proctoring maintain accepted standards? Telesurgeons generally maintain that if an operating surgeon takes special care to plan properly, takes the necessary precautions, and prepare contingencies in the event of a telecommunications failure, then the quality of instruction and procedural outcome should be at least as high as an ordinary training procedure. Indeed the operating surgeon must ensure that he is fully able to complete the procedure on his own before relying on telementoring.

As part of the planning process, the operating surgeon must send all relevant patient records to the telementor well in advance, providing enough time for him to thoroughly review and discuss the preoperative work up. The operating surgeon and his mentor must establish unequivocal rules of engagement[14] governing all conduct, procedures, and responsibilities for the operation based on a detailed preoperative review. Well before surgery begins, the two surgeons must prepare detailed contingency plans in the event of equipment failure or even total loss of communication. Such division of responsibility may prove difficult for surgeons to accept. "It is a considerable challenge for an experienced surgeon to yield this much control, even to a more experienced mentor; but it is critical to the safe performance of a procedure," James C. Rosser and colleagues have written as part of their telesurgical guidelines.[14]

Rosser et al. offer the following telesurgical guidelines:

Fully informed consent must be obtained from the patient. The experience of the operating surgeon and of the mentor must be candidly discussed and the risks, benefits, and alternatives thoroughly reviewed. . . . On the day of surgery, communication links should be established well before the patient enters the room. The mentor can then review the operating room setup with the circulating nurse and the scrub technician. The proper arrangement of personnel and equipment will ease the congestion in the room. This "pre-flight check list" will also assure that all the necessary equipment is present in the room, plugged in, and functioning well.

The mentor should be briefly introduced to the patient if possible. As the operation proceeds, the free flow of conversation must be somewhat limited and standardized to avoid confusion. The availability of a drawing device, the Surgistrator, allows the mentor to highlight relevant anatomy and impending targets or threats. A CD-ROM can supply video clips of the various steps in the procedure should there be a need for review during the case. Video tape "instant replay" allows the mentor to review events in the case and provide immediate feedback to the operating surgeon. Provision must be made for the mentor to see fluoroscopic or other diagnostic images obtained in the course of the case.

A debriefing session should be held after the case to review the conduct of the operation and telementoring experience. This will allow all of the participants to reflect on the experience and learn even more from it. Postoperatively, the mentor must be readily available and discussion of the patient's convalescence encouraged if the specter of the "teleitinerant surgeon" is to be avoided.[18]

As part of the division of procedural responsibility, other subtleties arise. From a financial perspective, physicians must ask: Who should be compensated for a telesurgical procedure? If a telemedical procedure is considered "experimental," will third party providers reimburse for it? Will the costs of advanced technologies in medicine fall as quickly as it has in other fields? What if costs remain high? Will telepresence create a new problem of teleitinerant surgeons?

To evaluate the feasibility of telementoring and teleproctoring, Rosser and John H. Payne performed a two-phase study.[15] In phase one, performed at the Detroit Riverside Hospital in Michigan during August 1994, surgeons augmented two-way audio-video communication with CD-ROM, instant-replay video monitoring, and a directional tool called a Surgistrator, that enables the telementor to indicate on the video monitor the points of entrance, dissection boundaries, and dangerous zones.

In phase two of the study, surgeons in Maastricht, The Netherlands, performed a telementored laparoscopic procedure, monitored by surgeons in Honolulu, Hawaii, through connections made via existing telephone lines and satellite links. Two cameras in Maastricht recorded the operation, one trained on the surgical team and the other on the laparoscope. Both surgeons, "half a world apart," experienced the same sounds and images nearly simultaneously, delayed by only 1.5 s (1500 msec). During this procedure the study's authors report that "16,000 kilometers and two oceans were shrunk to the dimension of a television monitor." Rosser and Payne state that they chose this "relatively routine" operation to "test the system while providing an extra margin of safety for the patient," focusing special attention on the synchrony and resolution of the two-way, real-time audio and video images.

In their evaluation Rosser and Payne reported that "the laparoscopic cholecystectomy in Maastricht was uneventful and quite successful. The surgeons were quite pleased with the experience. Numerous observers in both sites were also impressed with the technology and the potential of the concept. The patient was discharged in excellent condition on the second postoperative day." Despite the slight lag between sound, video image, and live action, the surgeons report that a "vivid interaction was possible."

The primary cost of setting up a suitable teleconferencing system for telementoring stems from telephone and satellite linkages. To connect surgeons in Maastricht and Honolulu with an ISDN-2 (Integrated Services Digital Network) line is modestly more expensive than an ordinary phone call, and far below that of an on-site mentoring or proctoring procedure, considering both the time and transportation costs involved. And as the expense of dedicated digital communications links—such as T1, T2, ISDN lines, which can rapidly transmit heavy digital loads—continues to fall, the quality and reliability of two-way video communication, and thus telesurgery, will improve.

In another feasibility test of telementored laparoscopy, Moore, Kavoussi,[19] and colleagues at the Johns Hopkins Bay View Medical Center evaluated 23 urology procedures. Located roughly 1000 feet from the operating room, an experienced surgeon remotely supervised a less experienced surgeon as he performed the procedure. The surgeons utilized two-way audio contact, real-time video relays, a robotic arm controlling the video-endoscope, and a telestrator. After comparing the telementored procedures with traditional side-by-side mentored surgery, the physicians concluded that in terms of outcomes, complications, and operative time, they considered the procedures successful. Indeed they reported an overall telementoring success rate of 95.6%—representing 22 of 23 procedures—with no increase in complications. In the one case of telementoring failure, a radical nephrectomy did not succeed due to improper positioning of the robotic arm. In terms of operative times, the surgeons found no statistical difference between traditional and telementored procedures for basic procedures, although in advanced cases telementoring took longer. Ultimately the surgical team concluded that the "telementoring of laparoscopic procedures is safe and feasible."

Medicine is only beginning to realize the possibilities of surgery and medical education at a distance. No longer do teacher and pupil, or proctor and trainee, have to work in the same location. The expert, or mentor, can transmit his or her expertise to remote areas where it would otherwise remain unavailable. The highest level of training can be maintained regardless of time or place. Teleconsultations can provide continuous, on-the-job training and lessen the isolation and insecurity of many physicians out in the field in small, rural communities.

In accepting the tremendous potentials and awesome responsibilities of new medical technologies, physicians and surgeons should consider the Statement on Telementoring and Teleproctoring issued by the Society of American Gastrointestinal and Endoscopic Surgeons.[20] This document offers prudent guidance: During initial implementation of new applications, only utilize such technologies under stringent protocols, which ensure patient safety and provide meaningful measures for outcome. All those who partake in this challenge should gauge their motives by a strict standard: Do such procedures truly benefit the patient?

III. TELEMEDICAL EDUCATION

General medical education, in addition to surgical training, is likely to benefit from simulators as standard teaching and reference tools.

To teach anatomy, Dr. Helene Hoffman of the University of California, San Diego,[21] has introduced virtual reality into an established multimedia computer education program. With this hybrid system students can learn pathology, radiology, and case studies from virtual anatomy—they can even practice medical and surgical procedures. For example, a student studying the gastrointestinal tract could "fly" into the stomach, observe an ulcer, and then biopsy it. This action could call up a histology micrograph of an ulcer, show a video tape of an ulcer operation, and predict healing response to medication. Since the virtual anatomy programs are run on a university network, students can access them from any location. They can even access the National Library of Medicine.

By virtue of such digital systems, the resources of education are now available to students without limitations on time, place, or schedule. Virtual reality serves in this system not only as an educational tool—for studying anatomy or practicing surgery—but also as a way to organize and display information.

For example, unlike a traditional library, where terms are indexed, the virtual cadaver serves itself as an index. Point to an organ or system in this virtual world and information about that organ appears. Data can be presented as text, X rays, histology sections, or video and audio clips. One learns from a virtual object the same way one learns in the real world: direct examination—pick up an object and look at it. Merging 3-D models with multimedia archival data transforms surgical education into a 4-D experience—three dimensions of space modified by one dimension of time.

To study the birthing process, for example, students and physicians can visualize and monitor labor and deliveries of newborns through the computer system of the Health Sciences Center at Brooklyn College in New York. This system facilitates the study of many documented cases and permits students to model scenarios from which they can learn.[22]

At the University of Pennsylvania, the Center for Human Modeling and Simulation is constructing 3-D representations of functional anatomy of organs and systems. For instance, in elucidating the respiratory system, the model demonstrates physiological changes such as pressure and flow, which change when subjected to anatomical deformations. Subsequently researchers will show how related systems interact with one another.[4]

Advanced technologies such as virtual environments may also permit students and researchers from around the world to attend, or even participate in, international medical conferences that they otherwise would miss, owing to the cost of travel or time away from the laboratory.

At East Carolina University, for example, more than 3000 educational programs, conferences, and meetings have been conducted over the medical school's telemedicine network since 1991, ranging from nursing courses and administrative meetings to weekly presentations of family medicine grand rounds to rural physicians.

V. SOCIOLOGICAL ISSUES AND TELEMEDICINE

Owing to social and behavioral patterns of the population at large, one tends to encounter from certain groups of physicians and patients—particularly the elderly or those uncomfortable with technology—a discomfort with, and even resistance to, the notion of telemedicine. Some patients balk at the "sterility" of their telemedical experiences and their uneasiness in interacting with a video monitor, declaring that they would rather have their doctor "with them."

However, while such attitudes hold firm for some individuals, in recent years there has been an evident shift in viewpoint of the general population toward greater acceptance of technology—and particularly of its use in medicine. One finds this trend notably true in three types of situations: First, where the alternative to telemedicine is no medicine at all; second, where individuals seem comfortable with a video technology, finding the experience natural and intuitive; third, where the telemedical experience appears so realistic that the patient is left with a feeling of personal presence.

In the first situation—where the alternative to telemedicine is no medicine—patients usually find themselves in remote, distant, or extreme environments. Examples of such locations include rural villages, prisons, expeditionary sites, or even a space station. On the one hand, patients may seem uncomfortable with the impersonality of video interactions; yet, on the other hand, they are grateful to have obtained medical care, which otherwise would have been unavailable.

In the second situation, a younger strata of patients are already comfortable with electronic interactions, even when medicine is involved. Having grown up in the Information Age, they feel at home with video monitors, telecommunications equipment, and virtual situations, finding such interactions to be quite natural and intuitive. In general, they see little problem with the practice of medicine at a distance, and some patients even seem to find the experience intriguing.

In the third situation, where the telemedical encounter feels extremely realistic, patients see the greatest potential for a powerful medical tool. As the technical ability to project a more realistic human improves, the relationship between patient and physician—even at a great distance—will feel more natural. Whereas televised pictures of distant lands, and even overseas telephone calls, once seemed so "faraway," today's technology increasingly creates the feeling that those distant figures are simply in the next room.

Two current research projects aim to achieve this effect using real-time 3-D representations. In one case Fuchs et al.[23] have mounted an array of CCD cameras on the walls and ceiling of a room, 3-D images to be transmitted back and forth between patients and physicians. To display these representations, Prince et al.[24] have designed a holographic system that projects free-standing models of a person into space. In theory, combining these technical feats will enable a physician to project a 3-D, lifelike, moving representation of a physician into a room with a patient at a distance, creating the illusion of actual presence.

Whether or not such representational methods in telemedicine prove cost effective, practical, or even desirable has not yet been determined. However, in the near future tools such as these will become available, thus enabling physicians to humanize, even personalize, telemedical interactions.

A variety of internet and media outlets have arisen to serve the high-tech needs of physicians and patients, including the Hospital Satellite Network, Cable Health Network, American Medical Television, and the United Medical Network. Moreover a web-site now exists for telemedicine information, called the Telemedicine Information Exchange (http://tie.telemed.org/). Through this web-site, a browser can download a wide variety of information, including journals, updates, reports, and technical details. The American Telemedicine Association has set up offices in northern Virginia to handle the growing needs of cybernautical health care professionals.

Moreover, the Telemedicine Research Center, a not-for-profit public service research corporation established in 1994 and based in Portland, Oregon, has dedicated itself to telemedicine research, education, and the creation, management and dissemination of information about telemedicine and telemedicine-related activities. The Center works in conjunction with the Clinical Telemedicine Cooperative Group.

VI. CONCLUSION

In the service of physician and patient responsibility, even skeptics should take a long view when evaluating the possible benefits of telemedical networks society. Telemedicine can potentially help treat a wide variety of illnesses affecting many sectors of society, both domestically and globally. To ensure an improvement in patient care, we must, as all medical technology advances, strive for "personalized" care in medicine for all patients.

Indeed the National Institute of Medicine's Committee on Evaluating Clinical Applications of Telemedicine drew the sober, even-handed conclusion that for some applications of telemedicine, more rigorous evaluations will make claims of their value more credible and will encourage their more widespread use. For other applications better evaluation may discourage adoption, at least until technologies or infrastructures improve or other circumstances change. This is to be expected. The purpose of evaluation—and the purpose of this report—is not to endorse telemedicine but to endorse the development and use of good information for decision making.

Yet, in keeping a skeptical view, one must not overlook the potential of telemedicine to help disadvantaged citizens obtain care that would be otherwise unattainable. Indeed telemedicine may promote the ultimate health care democracy—to make as much information and service available to as many people as possible, regardless of location or income.

REFERENCES

1. Field Marilyn J. ed.: Telemedicine: A Guide to Assessing Telecommunications in Health Care. Washington: National Academy Press, 1996:16.

2. Sanders JH, Tedesco FJ: "Telemedicine: Bringing medical care to isolated communities." *J Med Assoc Georgia* (May 1993):237–241.

3. Laplant A: "A virtual ER." Forbes ASAP (June 6, 1995):48–58.

4. Moline J: Virtual Environments for Healthcare: A White Paper for the Advanced Technology Program (ATP). Washington: National Institute of Standards and Technology, 1995:12.

5. Moline J: Virtual Environments for Healthcare: A White Paper for the Advanced Technology Program (ATP). Washington: National Institute of Standards and Technology, 1995:70.

6. Collins J: "Louisiana physician gears up for expanded tele-obstetrics." *Healthcare Telecom Report: The Newsletter of Communications and Information Systems Solutions* (Germantown, MD), April 10, 1995:1–2.

7. Balch DC, Tichenor JM: "Using telemedicine to expand the scope of health care information." *J Am Med Informa Assoc.* (Jan.–Feb. 1997), (4) 1:1–5.

8. Balch DC: "Telemedicine in rural North Carolina." *In Interactive Technology and the New Paradigm for Healthcare.* Washington: IOS Press, 1995:15–20.

9. Brecht R: 1995. Show report: Telemedicine 2000 highlights the state of the art in telemedicine, in Healthcare Telecom Report: The Newsletter of Communications and Information Systems Solutions (Germantown, MD), 3, 12 (June 5, 1995):8.

10. Wagner G: "As grant comes to a close, Iowa ponders future of DS-3 Telemedicine Network." In Healthcare Telecom Report: The Newsletter of Communications and Information Systems Solutions (Germantown, MD) 3, 12 (June 5, 1995):1–4.

11. Mecklenburg S: "Collaborative medicine comes to the High Plains via new network." In Healthcare Telecom Report: The Newsletter of Communications and Information Systems Solutions (Germantown, MD) 3, 10 (April 1995):3.

12. Western Governors' Association Telemedicine Action Report: 1995.

13. Perednia DA, Allen A: "Telemedicine technology and clinical applications." *J Am Med Assoc* (Feb. 8, 1995) 273:483–488.

14. Rosser JC: "Telementoring: A primer" (1995). Personal communication.

15. Go PMN, Payne JH, Satava RM, Rosser JC: "Teleconferencing bridges two oceans and shrinks the surgical world." In Zoltan S, Lewis JE, Fantini GA (eds.), Surgical Technology International IV. San Francisco: Universal Medical Press, 1995:29–31.

16. Kavoussi, LR: Site visit at the Urology Research Center, Bayview Medical Center, Johns Hopkins University, Baltimore, MD, February 1996.

17. Maresceaux J: Personal communication.

18. Satava RM: "Telementoring and teleproctoring for surgery," p. 2.

19. Kavoussi LR, Moore RG, Partin AW, Bender, JS, Zenilman ME, Satava RM: "Telerobotic assisted laparoscopic surgery: Initial laboratory and clinical experience." Urol 44:15–19, 1994.

20. SAGES Guidelines.

21. Hoffman H: "Developing network compatible instructional resources for UCSD's core curriculum." In Proc Medicine Meets Virtual Reality, San Diego, CA, June 1–2, 1992.

22. Brennan JP, Brennan JA: "Clinical applications of a high performance computing system for visualizing and monitoring human labor and birth." *In Interactive Technology and the New Paradigm for Healthcare.* Washington: IOS Press, 1995:48–52.

23. Fuchs: See of cameras.

24. Prince: DMA.

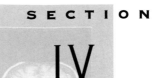
ETHICAL AND LEGAL CONSIDERATIONS

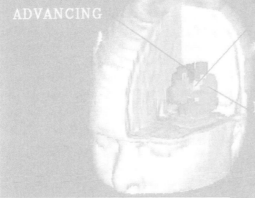

ADVANCING

STATIC

REGRESSING

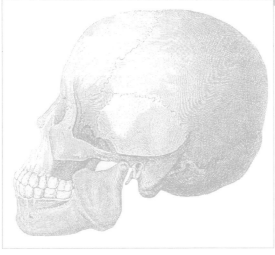

ETHICAL, LEGAL, AND MORAL ISSUES OF ADVANCED TECHNOLOGIES

KENNETH A. FORDE, M.D.

The world is wide
On every side
New wonders we can find.
And yet, for each man
Space extends
No farther than his mind.
　　　　—Anonymous

While the last two lines of this refrain suggest that the vision of the average individual is limited, the first three lines point out the broad imagination and ingenuity with which humankind is imbued. Robotics, telepresence surgery and virtual reality will probably prove to be but ripples in this boundless ocean of dreams and creativity.

The old adage "Necessity is the mother of invention" reminds us that creativity is often precipitated by need. If we assume that recent developments in these new technologies are tied to certain

Cybersurgery: Advanced Technologies for Surgical Practice,
Edited by Richard M. Satava, M.D.
ISBN 0-471-15874-7　Copyright © 1998 by Wiley-Liss, Inc.

current needs in our society, then the moral, legal, and ethical issues may be put in proper perspective. That, indeed, is the purpose of this chapter.

Among the current health care needs in our society are, on the one hand, the virtually global concern with reduction in cost and, on the other, the desire for wider availability of advanced medical technology. The concern with cost exists not only among the poorer countries but is equally present in those societies with a reputation for affluence. New medical technology and its dissemination are admittedly costly, and this expense is expected to increase for the foreseeable future. Could some of these costs be reduced and wider access achieved through the advanced technologies which are the subject of this book? Robotics, after all, offers the promise of decreasing the expense of operator fatigue, repetitive tasks, imprecision, physical proximity, and assisting personnel. Telepresence surgery may allow wider access to new technology limiting the need for travel by student, teacher and, sometimes by patient. Virtual reality, by combining three-dimensional imagery with the possibility of interactivity, offers the opportunity for improvement in surgical education and training through realistic computer simulation. Teaching may thus be easier, risks for patients less as new techniques are introduced and curtail the need for live animal research.[1] Also being developed are applications for complex medical database visualization and rehabilitation.[2]

Thus, while necessity may be the mother of invention, opportunity is often the father. Communications technology has proceeded apace with the availability of fiber-optic cables and satellites for image transmission with minimal delay. Its future seems unlimited as we approach the twenty-first century. It is therefore not surprising that those involved with the development of new technology are tempted and no doubt will "push the envelope" as far as is possible.

As the need and opportunity for this new technology is being translated to development and even implementation several issues have surfaced and will be discussed in this chapter. They include cost, access, behavior, legality, licensing, ownership, financing, security, evaluation, reimbursement, and effect on surgical training. These advanced technologies are still in the early stages of their evolution. The issues I raise will hardly be comprehensive, nor can I anticipate all the questions that need to be addressed. I hope merely to stimulate further engagement in the discussions surrounding these revolutionary advances in medicine. Most of the issues are interrelated and it will be difficult at times to separate them in discussion.

The interrelation of the topics under discussion is itself to be noted. What robotics, telepresence, and virtual reality have in common is that they represent *interventional* telemedicine. Hence the involvement of traditional interventionalists, namely surgeons. Telemedicine, defined in a variety of ways and with increasing interconnections with many traditional medical specialties (radiology, cardiology, and pathology) has been developed mainly in the areas of patient and physician education, consultation, and diagnosis.

I. COST

The development of television technology in the 1940s coupled with the launching of the Early Bird satellite two decades later led, not surprisingly, to demonstration projects funded, in the United States, by the federal government. The lull in interest in telemedicine that characterized the 1970s and 1980s had, in some part, to do with the fact that the technology was still in need of further development but was primarily due, as far as I can tell, to failure to come to reckoning with the next logical phase—the development of trial projects. The main stumbling block appeared to be cost, an element that still characterizes some of the current debate.

Despite the attractiveness of potential cost savings there is considerable skepticism about our ability to afford investment in these advanced technologies. Since the effectiveness and promise of these developments cannot be proved at this time, certain feasibility study expenses and start-up costs will have to be borne by government—in the United States at the federal level. Because of the over-whelming pressure to curb health care costs, with an ever more critical scrutiny of new medical technology, obtaining funding for such projects requires more lobbying than in former years. In the United States the Defense Emergency Supplemental and Recission Bill, the first such measure enacted in 1995, resulted in significant loss of funds for projects in various activities related to Telemedicine at the Departments of Commerce (including the National Telecommunications and Information Administration) and Defense (including the Defense Advanced Research Projects Agency). If Interventional Telemedicine is evaluated solely as the expansion of existing medical and surgical practice with computer and telecommunications technology, it is certainly not cost effective. However, it is entirely possible that by increasing access, improving training, and efficiency with enhanced outcome, this new technology could prove less costly to health care systems.

II. HUMAN BEHAVIOR

By a strict definition, "telemedicine" (medicine from a distance) is not new. In other times and cultures, for social or other reasons, the physician did not touch—sometimes did not look at the patient. Face-to-face contact between the patient and physician during a recognizable period of patient care has become the norm in our most advanced societies. Its potential erosion during adjustment to managed care in the United States has led to significant physician and patient concern. There are also legal implications of less than optimal care when such relationship cannot be amply demonstrated. How do we measure the importance to the surgical encounter of elements such as touch, feel, eye contact, and body language? Will we develop compensatory sensors? Will anxiety, fear, satisfaction, and confidence no longer be discernible in our patients?

III. SECURITY

Hard on the heels of this issue comes that of security, for the patient and for the physician. In this age of computers and expanded telecommunications, we have all become more exposed to new dimensions of technology. Identified commonly by universally registered and easily accessible codes, secrecy and confidentiality have been progressively eroded. In search of legal guidance for the medical staff, little is found. So far reliance has been placed on existing statutes governing traditional care. Since regulation of health care is largely a responsibility of state government, one looks to public agencies for guidance. A few states (notably Arkansas, California, Colorado, Louisiana) have established study commissions or appropriated funds for advanced medical issues. Among the few laws enacted is Colorado's HB1272, which indicates that persons practicing on individuals residing in Colorado will be deemed to be practicing medicine in that state, regardless of the practitioner's location. Given the use of computers and telecommunication, data acquisition and modification are certainly possible. In order to protect the patient, the physician issues to be addressed include unwarranted and inappropriate disclosure, data manipulation, tampering, or unplanned destruction. Perpetrators of such adverse acts may be insiders (personnel) or outsiders (computer "hackers"). Potential solutions include staff training, identification of the type of information that might be most sensitive to patients, physical controls, use of passwords, differing levels of access, signed confidentiality agreements, policies for correcting or destroying records and for monitoring compliance with security regulations.

With the expanding development and use of the Internet conflicts between print and electronic journalism are being discussed. The same will doubtless hold true for all forms of information. For example, who owns information?[3]

IV. LEGAL ISSUES

This and the questions of security will also come to bear on the issue of litigation. This places much onus on state governments. In the United States malpractice actions often have as a basis the presumed or alleged deviation of the physician from standard practice, which varies from state to state. Current case law regards the patient and physician in the telemedicine experience to have established a doctor-patient relationship and thus subject to laws governing such relationships in a particular state. In specific cases courts have determined that contractual obligations to the patient exist: If the consultant has met or knows the patient by name, if the consultant has examined the patient's records, if the consultant has accepted a fee for services rendered.[4] Since telemedicine arrangements may involve more than one state, it is possible that potential plaintiffs and their lawyers may shop for what would appear to be the most favorable jurisdictions for them. Another question being asked by attorneys is: Are there risks inherent in the technology itself? For example, does the lack of person-to-person, face-to-face contact reduce the accuracy of the physician's evaluation? Does data compression reduce the quality of information and, especially, endoscopic images. Will the practitioner be liable for errors related to delays in transmission or equipment failure? How can informed consent be properly obtained?

V. LICENSURE

Issues of credentialling and licensure also have liability relevance, and since (1) the license to practice medicine is issued by states and (2) telemedicine will often be practiced across state lines, the Federation of State Medical Boards of the United States, Inc.[5] which has been studying these questions has drafted "An Act to Regulate the Practice of Medicine across State Lines." The model act calls for an abbreviated licensure process to be administered by the patient's state of residence. One of the consequences of this proposed legislation would be to obligate the telemedicine practitioner to the regulations of the Medical Practice Act in the particular state, including surrender of records when requested, subject to disciplinary action if deemed necessary by that state's medical board, and to follow the confidentiality requirements of that state.

By now the reader should realize that much of the legislation proposed or enacted, for all practical purposes, has to do primarily with education, diagnostic, and consultative telemedicine. Even so, it is still limited and in the exploratory phase. In some ways it is fortunate that the areas of robotics, telepresence, and virtual reality are still not fully developed and ubiquitous, for many of the considerations in this book are still in the infancy of concern and discussion.

VI. EVALUATION

However, several groups of scientists are working on methods of evaluating telemedicine for safety and efficiency through laboratory experimentation as well as clinical utility and effectiveness through large field trials.[6,7] While this type of research characterizes the biomedical world and properly is concerned with accuracy, reliability, precision, sensitivity, and specificity, those responsible for health care delivery must focus on acceptance and effects of advanced technology. The concerns here will be accessibility, quality, and cost and the perspectives of the patient, the provider, and society. Studies will have to be detailed, evaluating such basic elements as effects on timing and accuracy of diagnosis, efficiency of patient flow, and disease outcomes. Patients will have to be evaluated for not only satisfaction but for access to care, knowledge, and attitude about condition. Managed care providers will doubtless be interested in these elements as well as patient load and mix, while institutions will look at productivity, efficiency, and reimbursement. The community as a whole will have to concern itself with issues of availability, affordability, and cost-sharing or substitution in comparison with other resources. It is the recognition of these multifactorial issues that has led the leaders of organizations such as the Society of American Gastrointestinal Endoscopic Surgeons (SAGES) to advise that the enthusiasm for advanced technology be tempered by orderliness and restraint.[8]

VII. SURGICAL TRAINING

SAGES and other organizations that are concerned with surgical education and training must also be concerned that training in advanced technology is conducted in a fashion that will provide for safe and efficient patient care. The SAGES Framework for Post-Residency Surgical Education and Training[9] addresses the relevant issues in a comprehensive manner but, like any such document, may need revision to include elements of more advanced technology as it becomes available. As this technology becomes more fully developed we must ask: Does it have the potential for decreasing the duration and therefore the cost of training future surgeons? Could the surgical trainee of the twenty-first century graduate or be certified having performed fewer procedures, since they could be learned later through a telementoring postgraduate program?

Those responsible for the training and certification of surgeons, have held that in addition to the development of technical skills, a surgeon should exercise mature judgment and should have been observed by those responsible for the inculcation of surgical skills over a period of time.

VIII. CONCLUSION

This has been but a brief foray into the ethical, legal, and moral issues in the debate over the place of the advanced surgical technology of robotics, telepresence, and virtual reality in health care—

what, for want of a unifying concept, I have called and discussed under the generic term "interventional telemedicine." Perhaps Fielding put it best: "Clearly these innovations are intended to benefit the patients, and therefore we must consider what is in the public interest. We must also recognize that although the benefits and risks are describable by the physician, they are in fact borne by the individual patient undergoing the procedure."[10]

REFERENCES

1. Satava RM: "Virtual reality surgical simulation." *Surg Endosc* (1993) 7:203–205.

2. Satava RM: "Medical applications of virtual reality." *J Med Systems* (1995) 19:275–280.

3. Branscomb AW: Who Owns Information? From Privacy to Public Access. New York: Basic Books, 1994.

4. Granade PF: "Malpractice issues in the practice of telemedicine." *Telemed J* (1995) 1:87–89.

5. Federation of State Medical Boards of the United States, Inc., 400 Fuller Wiser Road, Eules, TX 76039–3855.

6. Perednia DA. "Telemedicine system evaluation and a collaborative model for multi-centered research." *J Med Systems* (1995) 19:287–294.

7. Tangalos EG: Clinical Trials to validate Telemedicine. *J Med Syst* (1995) 19:281–185.

8. SAGES: "Statement on telementoring and teleproctoring." *Surg Endosc* (1995) 9:1037.

9. SAGES: "Framework for post-residency surgical education and training." SAGES Guideline. *Surg Endosc* (1994) 8:1137–1142.

10. Fielding IP: "Philosophical considerations in laparoscopic coloproctology." In Arregui ME, Sackier JM (eds.), Minimal Access Coloproctology. Oxford and New York: Radcliffe Medical Press, 1995:217–224.

INDEX